D0359909

Same-Sex Attraction

Same-Sex Attraction
A Parents' Guide

Edited by
John F. Harvey, OSFS, & Gerard V. Bradley

ST. AUGUSTINE'S PRESS
South Bend, Indiana
2003

Manufactured in the United States of America.

1 2 3 4 5 6   09 08 07 06 05 04 03

Library of Congress Cataloging in Publication Data
Same-sex attraction: a parents' guide / edited by John F. Harvey
    and Gerard V. Bradley.
        p. cm.
    ISBN 1-58731-751-6 (hardcover : perm. paper)
    1. Homosexuality – Religious aspects. 2. Homosexuality – Moral
    and ethical aspects. 3. Sexual ethics. I. Harvey, John F. (John
    Francis), 1918– II. Bradley, Gerard V., 1954–
    BL65.H64 S26 2002
    24'.66 – dc21   2002012095

∞ *The paper used in this publication meets the minimum requirements of the*
American National Standard for Information Sciences - Permanence of Paper
for Printed Materials, ANSI Z39.48-1984.

Contents

Appendices

Introduction

Beginning in February 1998, Professor Gerard Bradley of Notre Dame Law School and I, Father John Harvey OSFS, weighed the need for a book which parents of persons with *same-sex* attractions could read to understand the nature of the homosexual condition and the immorality of homogenital acts. We came to believe that such parents would welcome contributions from scholars on the complex issues involved in homosexuality and the homosexual movement. Accordingly, we have chosen scholars in Holy Scripture, Dogmatic and Moral Theology, Philosophy, Canon and Civil Law, Pastoral Theology, Psychology and Psychiatry. The impact of the gay movement on marriage and family life is discussed in terms of its limitations on the freedom of conscience of both individuals and institutions which reject homogenital behavior as immoral. Several authors stress the necessity of providing guidance to parents and families in caring for their sons or daughters who have *same-sex* attractions.

Helen Hull Hitchcock, mother of four daughters and director and founder of Women for Faith and Family, opens the volume with a brief meditation on the confusion and anxiety experienced by both the parents and the child with *same-sex* attractions, at whatever stage of growth.

In our "Science" section, Dr. Jeffrey Satinover unfolds the biological truth about homosexuality. Satinover shows that the so-called "gay gene" – ordaining certain people to a homosexual lifestyle – is a myth.

Dr. Joseph Nicolosi follows with his insightful description of viewing 'gay' as a "self-deceptive identity . . . seized upon by an individual," and increasingly supported by our society, in order to solve emotional conflicts.

A distinguished canonist, Monsignor Cormac Burke, explains the relationship between the canonical validity of a marriage and recent developments in psychology and psychiatry concerning the homosexual condition. He is concerned with the confusion about homosexuality generated by the ego-syntonic mentality (the "learning to like oneself" approach) that has dominated psychological thought and therapeutic practice for the last fifty years. He suggests that man should consider the advice of Pope John Paul II in *Veritatis Splendor:* "I ask everyone to look more deeply at man, whom Christ has saved in the mystery of his love, and at the human being's unceasing search for truth and meaning."

Dr. Kevin Miller has the lead chapter in the "Morality" section. He takes readers into the complexities of scriptural analysis. He explains clearly the interrelationship of Divine Oral Tradition and Holy Scripture, as the Church has used them to contradict revisionist interpretations, and to affirm that we have a vocation to chastity in Christ – a vocation that is incompatible with homosexual acts.

One of the Church's great moral theologians, Father Benedict Ashley, O.P., discusses the "Theology of Hetero- and Homosexuality." Fr. Ashley reaffirms the conclusions of Professor Kevin Miller – that all are called to chastity – and uses Aquinas in his repudiation of the false teaching that persons with *same-sex* attractions should live in a "stable *same-sex* partnership." Ashley adds that through a life of celibacy out of love of God the "homosexual condition can become the occasion of a great good."

Dr. John Finnis, philosopher, theologian, and jurist, addresses the misunderstanding in the minds of many Catholics on the meaning of the term, "objective disorder." He says that "the reason why even the most deep-seated homosexual tendency must be called disordered is straightforward. Every such tendency, inclination, or orientation 'is a more or less strong tendency ordered toward an intrinsic moral evil.'" Finnis also argues from the nature of human sexuality and marriage to the intrinsic evil of homosexual acts. He points out that the very term "sexual orientation" is radically equivocal – a point that helps us understand the confusion found in gay-rights legislation.

The matter of *same-sex* unions and "marriages" is addressed by Cardinals Bevilacqua and O'Connor and by Professor Gerard Bradley of the University of Notre Dame Law School. Cardinal Bevilacqua's testimony before the City Council of Philadelphia eloquently explains the necessary involvement of the Church in an issue that directly attacks marriage and family life. It is not unjust discrimination to support the institution of marriage, and not to legalize same-sex partnerships or same-sex "marriages."

Cardinal O'Connor argues that the legalization of *same-sex* marriage would equate the non-married state with the married state. This cannot fail to influence the young in their attitudes toward marriage and the family, "even discouraging marriage in instances when marriage should be encouraged." Indirectly but truly, such legislation will weaken the most important building block of a well ordered society, the family. For its own sake, civil government must do all it can to protect the family from same-sex marriage legislation.

Gerard Bradley criticizes the various arguments proposed by advocates of same-sex marriage. He sees these arguments as lacking a definition of marriage, as it has been found in cultures throughout the centuries. He says that "contemporary common sense, as well as our legal and moral traditions, point us to the existence of some decisive relation among marriage, children, and how children come to be. The practical insight that marriage has its own intelligible point and that it is a one flesh communion of persons consummated and actualized in the reproductive-type acts of spouses, cannot be attained by someone who has no idea of what these terms mean, nor can it be attained, except by strenuous efforts of the imagination, by people who, due to personal circumstance, have little acquaintance with actual marriages thus understood."

In the pastoral section Helen Hull Hitchcock reviews how the Protestant Churches have developed programs for persons with same-sex attractions. There are great differences among them. She also describes and criticizes many groups within the Catholic Church who are not faithful to the teachings of the Church.

Alan P. Medinger focuses on homosexuality as a false identity. The title of his essay is: "Calling Oneself 'Gay' or 'Lesbian' Clouds One's Self-Perception." Medinger understands the pain and confusion of parents when their sons and daughters come home at Christmas break, proclaiming that they are "gay" or "lesbian." Young men and women are easily seduced by the powerful gay lobbies on college campuses. They begin to believe that the gay lifestyle alone will make them happy. The longer one remains in this lifestyle, the more deeply one's false identity is imbedded. From his own life experience of change of identity, Medinger affirms that many more have been able to come out of the false identity. It is not an easy process, but with the help of God, it can take place.

In this, the pastoral section of this volume, I provide a 'Question and Answer' section for parents of children with same-sex attractions. It is based upon the many communications I have had with such parents and, like Medinger, I have tried to help them handle their grief. While Courage has had programs for parents since 1990 – called EnCourage – we need to develop a better program for them.

Included as an appendix is the text of a document issued in the name of the National Conference of Catholic Bishops' Committee on Marriage and Family, called *Always Our Children (Revised)*. In this paper some bishops sought to address much the same problem that we do: how to enlighten and pastorally guide parents of children with same-sex attractions. In response to concerns expressed by the Vatican, the original text of *Always Our Children* (1997) was superseded (July 1998) by the text printed here. A critique of *AOC (Revised)*, by me, concludes this book.

Rev. John F. Harvey, OSFS
Director of Courage
April, 2002

What Will Become of Our Children?
Helen Hull Hitchcock

Rachel is a single mother of a fourteen-year-old son, Alan. Rachel, a faithful Catholic in her late thirties, was abandoned by Alan's father before her only child's birth. The boy became the center of Rachel's life. She has done her best to raise him – with scarce money from welfare, part-time jobs, and her parents. Even though it meant she could not have an outside job, Rachel was an "at-home mom" until Alan started kindergarten in their small midwestern town. Even when she got a part-time job, she made sure she would be there when Alan came home from school.

Rachel was determined that Alan would have a solid, normal upbringing, despite the absence of his father. She thanked God that her son was healthy and bright, energetic and blessed with a sunny, affectionate disposition. One of Rachel's greatest consolations has been that, even as a small child, Alan showed an unusual interest in his religion. He loved the Bible stories she read him; he learned his prayers and never failed to say them. He seemed to take real interest in his classes in preparation for Confirmation two years ago. Even now, he never whines about going to church.

Rachel's parents, who live across town, are a great help to her. Rachel's father, a retired teacher, is especially fond of Alan. Well aware of the boy's need for a father, he has done his best to assume that role. He even quit smoking in order to set a good example for Alan (who, unlike most of his friends, never took up the habit).

Lately, Rachel has been worried about Alan. Last year he did poorly in school, and begged not to have to ride the school bus, saying that he had become the victim of cruel teasing by some of the older boys. So this year Rachel transferred him to a school in a nearby small town, which involved a ten-mile drive each way every day. She thought things were better, at least at first. But Alan was changing – physically and in other ways Rachel couldn't quite explain. He often seemed silent and sullen. When he came home from school, he mostly played video games or "surfed the 'net." If Rachel asked about school, he just grunted. He seemed to be losing interest in everything but the computer screen. He was neglecting his homework, and his grades were slipping again. She reminded herself that confusion and changes were to be expected in adolescents, and tried not to worry too much.

This afternoon, while Rachel was busy sorting laundry in the kitchen, Alan walked in and stood beside the laundry basket. Rachel looked up and saw his eyes were filled with tears. Before she could ask him what was wrong, Alan blurted out, "Mom, I have to tell you. I'm gay."

This story is fictional, but it is typical. There are too many Rachels weeping for their children, and too many confused Alans. We know them. We have heard their cries for help. How can we help parents of youngsters like Alan? What can be done to help people like Rachel and Alan and their families? What can we do to change attitudes and overcome forces within our society which so jeopardize families and children, and thus the future of society? What about the churches? What should the Catholic Church be doing?

This volume answers these questions.

Science

The Biological Truth about Homosexuality
Jeffrey Satinover

The cultural and legal conflict over homosexuality is fraught with unrecognized confusion because it rests, in part, on concepts and findings from a new and extremely complex branch of science – the genetics of human behavior. The overarching goal of behavioral genetics is to clarify the relationship between nurture and nature in human life. This, however, has been an area of concern for philosophers and theologians since time immemorial. We should not be surprised, therefore, that a science that encompasses such complicated questions is hard to grasp and easy to distort. Behind gay politics is "gay science." Behind gay politics, in other words, is the manipulation of scientific knowledge in support of the *moral* legitimization and *legalization* of homosexuality and the so-called gay lifestyle.

In today's relentless barrage of words, images, slogans, and ideas that assault us from all sides, many of us have become dependent on sound bites – short, simple, predigested, emotion-laden, one-stop conclusions. We have neither the time nor the ability to sort through the primary information for ourselves in order to arrive at our own considered conclusions. As a result, the deep complexity of the scientific research into homosexuality is easy for people to misinterpret and easier still to misuse.

Here is one example.

On July 15, 1993, National Public Radio reported a new study in *Science* due to be released the next day. The tenor of the report was to celebrate the so-called discovery of the gene that causes homosexuality. Near the end, the necessary caveats were quickly added, but most laymen would have turned off the radio thinking that homosexuality is genetically determined.

Print media reinforced this impression. The *Wall Street Journal* headlined their report the next day, "Research Points Towards a Gay Gene." A subheading of the *Journal* article stated "Normal Variation," leaving the casual reader with the impression that the research led to this conclusion. It did not, nor could it have. In fact, the subhead merely alluded to nothing more than the researchers' personal, unsubstantiated *opinions* that homosexuality, as they put it, "is a normal variant of human behavior." Even the *New York Times*, in its more moderate front-page article, "Report Suggests Homosexuality Is Linked to Genes," noted that researchers warned against overinterpreting the work, "or taking it to mean anything as simplistic as that the 'gay gene' had been found." At the end of the *Wall Street Journal* article, at the bottom of the last paragraph on the last page deep within the paper, a prominent geneticist was quoted for his reactions to the research. He observed that "the gene . . . may be involved in something other than sexual behavior. For example, it may be that the supposed gene is only 'associated' with homosexuality, rather than a 'cause' of it." This rather cryptic comment would be difficult to understand without the needed background information. Yet it is the most critical distinction in the article.

To disentangle this confusion – and to form solid principles by which to reach responsible conclusions – requires effort. But readers who persist and grasp the basic truths about the science of human behavior will gain an invaluable insight into the debate over homosexuality. And these readers, whether politicians, educators, clergy, mental health professionals, or concerned parents, will also understand how limited are science's answers to questions of right and wrong. We will find, too, that when we reach the proper limits of science, we have to leave science behind to proceed further.

I

The Genetic Contribution to Homosexuality

One way to simplify and begin to approach the complex question of the genetic contribution to homosexuality is to consider that the genetic contribution to *any* trait need not be direct; actually, when the trait is behavioral, the genetic contribution is usually *not* direct. In other words genes often contribute to some other phenomenon that in turn *facilitates* some behavioral patterns and makes others less likely, yet determines none.

An obvious example of this principle is basketball. No genes exist that code for becoming a basketball player. But some genes code for height and the elements of athleticism, such as quick reflexes, favorable bone structure, height-to-weight ratio, muscle strength and refresh rate, metabolism and energy efficiency, and so on. Many such traits have racial distributions (which makes the genetic connection evident), resulting in more men of Bantu or Nordic stock (being taller) playing on professional basketball teams than men of Pygmy or Appenseller-Swiss stock (being shorter).

Someone born with a favorable (for basketball) combination of height and athleticism is in no way genetically programmed or forced to become a basketball player. These qualities, however, certainly facilitate that way of life. As a consequence basketball playing has a clear genetic component, due to the hereditability of height. Were scientists to undertake a study of basketball-playing comparable to the studies that have been done to date on the genetics of homosexuality, they would find a much higher degree of apparent genetic influence than for homosexuality. But even in the case of basketball, the comparatively stronger genetic correlation does not mean that people are forced to play basketball.

What do we know about biology and homosexuality? We can summarize the conclusions about the biology of homosexuality in ten points.

First, a certain genetic constitution may make homosexuality more readily available as a life course – hence statistically more likely – but it is not a cause of homosexuality. Without that constitution later homosexuality is less likely. This is the same *general* conclusion we reached for basketball, though (as I said) the genetic component of basketball playing is much greater than it is for homosexuality.

Second, *if* we accept proponents' research at *face value*, this predisposition contributes no more than 25 to 50 percent to the likelihood of an individual actually becoming homosexual. But a more critical, realistic assessment of the research shows that the genetic contribution, though not zero, is likely to turn out to be far smaller than that – perhaps between 10 percent and 25 percent.

Third, when the actual incidence of homosexuality in a population is higher, the apparent influence of this possible genetic predisposition will be lesser, and the influence of non-genetic factors greater. For example, if a trait is almost universal, two genetically identical twins are just as likely to share it as are two unrelated individuals. On the other hand, if the trait is extremely rare, the twins will likely share it only if they share some important factor common to both (such as a gene or genes, or environment).

Fourth, the incidence of homosexuality depends on its definition. In some cultures, in certain classes, sexual relations between older men and adolescents is ubiquitous. Activists routinely appeal to such cultures as an argument for the "normality" of homosexuality – considering such relations as just that: evidence of homosexuality. In such cultures the genetic contribution to homosexuality is zero. In short, if the incidence of homosexuality is great, and there are cultures where it is nearly universal (as activists argue), then the studies that purport to show it being genetic are 100 percent meaningless.

In fact, there is a huge cultural variability in incidence – from 1 to 100 percent at the extremes – and this suggests the possibility that there are many different strains of homosexuality. At a minimum two strains exist: one strain linked indirectly to a complex genetic component of the limited sort previously discussed, such as in the relationship of height to basketball-playing; the other would be almost entirely influenced by culture. The former would tend to be present in some measure even when culturally taboo and would be associated with a very low incidence rate. The latter would predominate in cultures where the taboos against homosexuality were nonexistent or relatively weak and would be associated with a relatively high incidence rate. In cultures such as ours where the taboo is weakening there is likely to be a mixture of types present.

Fifth, given that cultures have existed where the incidence of homosexuality is far greater – or lower – than presently in our culture, the incidence of homosexuality is clearly influenced by mores. Where people endorse and encourage homosexuality, the incidence increases; where they reject it, it decreases. These factors have nothing to do with its genetics. One occasionally hears the claim that these cultural variations in the incidence of homosexuality are illusions, that in fact, there has been a rather steady incidence across cultures and through history. There is *no* evidence to support this claim, which usually rests upon dogmatic *belief* in strict genetic causation of homosexuality. In fact, there is no reason to discount or ignore the abundant evidence that different societies experience sharply different rates of homosexuality.

Sixth, some yet-to-be-determined proportion of any apparent genetic influence on homosexuality is actually a non-genetic, though innate, prenatal influence. This influence may be hormonal, autoimmune, from some undiscovered factor or factors, or a combination of all these. The proportion of this seemingly genetic but actually intrauterine and non-genetic influence is neither "all" nor "none." It may well be closer to the former than the latter if certain European studies on hormonal effects prove correct. This intrauterine influence may be an abnormality that could eventually prove to be correctable. Nonetheless, the practical influence of such an intrauterine predisposition can be at most no more than the maximum degree of seeming heritability – that is, considerably less than 50 percent – since none of the studies to date can tell the difference between them.

Seventh, of the remaining 50 to 90 percent of the extrauterine, non-innate causes of homosexuality, a substantial but not yet quantifiable portion represents the individual's response to both environmentally reinforced attitudes and behaviors as well as to innate pre-dispositional pressures.

Eighth, whatever genetic contribution to homosexuality exists, it probably contributes not to homosexuality *per se*, but rather to some other trait that makes the homosexual option more readily available than to those who lack this genetic trait (as in the correlation between height and basketball). The homosexual option may be selected for personal reasons, such as a response to trauma, or social reasons, such as overcrowding, sub-cultural mores, or both. It is reinforced each time it is selected. Therefore it is even more likely to be re-selected the next time.

Ninth, in light of population genetics and the importance of replacement rates, the fact that homosexuality continues to exist suggests strongly that: (1) genetic influences are far from sufficient to cause homosexuality, though they may increase its likelihood; (2) the genes that influence the appearance of homosexuality do not code for homosexuality per se, but rather for other traits that themselves do not adversely affect heterosexual reproduction.

And tenth, most studies to date have many flaws. Some are caused by the intrusion of political agendas into what should be objective research, and some are due to the complex nature of the subject. These flaws must temper any conclusions we make. It is premature (and will almost certainly prove to be incorrect) simply to state that homosexuality "is" or "is not" genetic, innate, psychological, chosen, or social. It was extremely premature to pronounce, decades ago, that homosexuality is not a psychological illness.

II
Non-genetic Influences upon Human Behavior

My primary aim has been to demonstrate that hard science is far from providing an explanation of homosexuality, let alone one that reduces it to genetic determinism. My purpose so far will have been well served if the discussion helps to guard against the grossly overblown claims of interest groups who misuse science for political ends. As we have seen in the case of homosexuality, for all the public fanfare, science has accomplished almost nothing we did not know from common sense: One's character traits are in part innate but are subject to modification by experience and choice.

Before we examine these non-genetic influences on homosexuality we will look at the classic example of a similar phenomenon in the area of behavioral *problems* – alcoholism – and at some of the still tentative theories that are emerging to explain it.

It has long seemed that problem drinking has a genetic component. Even after social and family influences have been taken into account, evidence remains that when a gene or set of genes are present in an individual or family there is a much higher risk for serious alcoholism. Furthermore, certain national and transnational gene pools (Irish, Scandinavian, Northern European in general) seem to be predisposed to alcoholism.

It turns out that the genetic makeup of Northern Europeans' nervous systems are more "high strung"; Northern Europeans react (on average) with an intense nervous system arousal to a perceived threat. This is experienced subjectively as anxiety; alcohol is the original anti-anxiety agent. People with this predisposition to intense anxiety responses are therefore more likely to find their way into greater alcohol use because for them alcohol gives a greater degree of emotional relief than it does to the more laid-back "Mediterranean" type.

Why might Northerners have this disposition in greater proportion than Southerners? The answer may lie not so much in the distinction between "north" and "south" or even "warm" and "cold," as in "Polar" versus "Equatorial." At issue is not the location itself but the differing cycles of light found close to and far from the equator. The harsher climate and reduced intensity of light found nearer the poles is not only associated with differences in body build and skin color but also with differences in the nervous system. The northern races have adapted to the harshness of their environment by developing more easily stimulated nervous systems than have the equatorial races.

In its pure form, this genetic type not only reacts subjectively, but also responds to stresses with intense physiologic responses such as increased heart rate and blood pressure, skin flushing, perspiring palms and soles, and so on. All these responses, subjective and physiologic, are mediated by the nervous system. Alcohol calms all of these by soothing the underlying nerves.

Thus genetics strongly predisposes individuals toward alcoholism. And yet no genes specifically code for it. This seeming contradiction can be explained by the fact that some genes do code for the anxiety response, and under certain circumstances an especially intense response is adaptive. Those who carry such genes may be more likely to develop alcoholism than those who do not carry them. This does not mean, however, that alcoholism is itself directly genetic, natural, and a good thing (as activists claim of homosexuality) – nor that it is an illness in the strict sense of the word.

Of interest in comparing alcoholism to homosexuality is the fact that alcoholism is estimated to be between 50 percent and 60 percent heritable; homosexuality to be less than 50 percent even by activists, probably considerably less. This even greater risk for alcoholism does not lead to the conclusion, however, that alcoholics are not responsible for controlling, changing, or stopping the behavior.

The analogy between, on the one side, alcoholism and anxiety and, on the other, homosexuality and some unknown intermediate trait, may be more than an analogy. For there is evidence that unusually intense anxiety responses are also associated with an increased tendency toward homosexuality.

III
Non-genetic Influences upon Homosexuality

If homosexuality is not entirely genetic in origin, where does it come from? If homosexuality were in fact directly genetic, and thus present in some form from birth (and before), it would likely be associated with an early onset of some form of "homosexual identity." But this presents an implicit conundrum, for homosexuality is associated with far lower childbearing rates than is heterosexuality. At present, and for the past thirty years, the childbearing rate for the United States as a whole has hovered around 1.05 children per adult. But 1.05 happens also to be the minimum "replacement" rate.

Because the total American rate is an average of the rate for both heterosexuals and homosexuals, the homosexual rate must therefore be considerably lower than the replacement rate. To whatever extent that homosexuality is significantly and directly genetic – and thus homosexuals would mostly discover their "orientation" prior to marriage – its presence in the population would shrink from one generation to the next. Unless it were continuously "redeveloped" by some nonheritable cause or causes, intrauterine or otherwise, it would eventually disappear.

The fact that the incidence of homosexuality does not appear to be declining – a point the activists emphasize – is thus itself an argument *against* it being *directly* genetically determined. This argument would not hold if genes that merely indirectly increased the likelihood of homosexuality were directly associated with some other trait that enhanced survival and reproduction.

It is much easier to ask the meaningless, but subtly bias-inducing, sound-bite question, "Isn't homosexuality genetic?" than to ask the much more realistic – but frustratingly complex – question, "To what degree is homosexuality (or any other behavioral trait) genetic and non-genetic, innate and acquired, familial and non-familial, intrauterine-influenced and extrauterine-influenced, affected by the environment and independent of the environment, responsive to social cues and unresponsive to these cues, and when and in what sequence do these various influences emerge to generate their effects and how do they interact with one another; and after we have put these all together, how much is left over to attribute to choice, repetition, and habit?"

The non-genetic factors that can influence the development of a behavioral pattern fall into five categories:

1. Intrauterine (prenatal) effects, such as the hormonal milieu (environment);

2. Extrauterine (postnatal) physical effects, such as trauma, viruses;

3. Extrauterine "symbolic" effects, such as familial interactions, education;

4. Extrauterine experience, such as the reinforcing effect of the repetition of behaviors;

5. Choice.

IV
Intrauterine Influences

The lack of 100 percent similarity for sexual orientation of identical twins shows that the non-genetic factor(s) influencing homosexuality cannot be *exclusively* intrauterine. If they were, then the concordance rate for homosexuality would be nearly 100 percent – because identical twins share the same prenatal environment. In fact, if there are any intrauterine effects, they would contribute to the 50 percent *apparently genetic* effect (concordance) that was described earlier. Once these factors were identified and segregated out, the actual remaining genetic effect would be that much smaller.

But a vast body of research has emerged over the past decade that demonstrates how biological factors powerfully influence brain development. These factors therefore affect cognitive, emotional, and behavioral expression, and so, at least in principle, may contribute to homosexuality. Even small differences between individuals will result in statistically significant average differences between two large populations. But, unexpectedly, the most powerful effects on male-versus-female brain development do not occur directly from male-versus-female *genetic* differences, but indirectly by way of the maternal intrauterine hormonal milieu.

Put simply, the hormonal environment in which a baby develops is a balance of androgenic (male) and estrogenic (female) hormones. A genetically male baby signals the mother to generate a more heavily androgenic environment than does a female baby. The particular hormonal balance then determines whether the baby will develop typically male or typically female genitalia, bodily characteristics, and brain structures.

Because the maternal hormonal response varies, the masculinizing or feminizing influences are different for each developing baby. There is a large degree of overlap between men and women with respect to the brain. The secondary sexual characteristics (genitalia), however, take only two distinct forms, except in very unusual circumstances. That is to say, though everyone (practically speaking) is either male or female by virtue of their reproductive organs, we are all somewhat of a "mix" in terms of brain development. Let me explain.

In spite of the obvious general differences between men and women, a great many men have somewhat feminine physical features and a great many women have somewhat masculine features, all well within normal. Many women are actually more masculine than many men, and many men are actually more feminine than many women; yet all these, too, are well within normal. Furthermore, some women are more masculine than the average man, and some men are more feminine than the average woman, and these are also entirely normal. And yet it remains true that on average (which is to say, as a group), women are more feminine than men and men are more masculine than women. These differences should therefore show up in the average differences in behavior between the two groups.

To a less obvious but significant degree, these statistical differences extend to brain development as well. Thus the cognitive, emotional, and behavioral expressions of the male and female classes as a whole are affected to various degrees by masculine and feminine influences. Again, there is much overlap. Therefore many normal men have rather more feminine behavioral characteristics, and many normal women have rather more masculine behavioral characteristics. Little of this overlap, however, predicts homosexuality.

From time to time the chemical signals get crossed. The maternal hormonal milieu of, for example, a genetically male baby will then be very far to the feminine end of the spectrum. In these unfortunate cases, her genitalia, body type, brain, and behavior will develop physically as a normal-appearing female. She remains, however, genetically male and therefore infertile. We conventionally refer to such individuals according to their body type and not their genetic makeup, because they will live according to the former.

(In rare cases, the milieu is ambiguous. Regardless of the baby's genetic structure, the baby will emerge a hermaphrodite – one with variable proportions of male and female features. The parents will be obliged to choose a sex for their child to be defined surgically, which may or may not correspond to the genetic background.)

Clearly, then, an important determinant of at least certain behavioral predispositions is the hormonal environment. Thus, some proportion of what appears to be genetic in homosexual behavior may actually be a nongenetic intrauterine effect on the parts of the brain that influence sexual behavior.

V

The Role of the Family and Childhood Trauma

One of the most consistent findings from the studies of homosexuality is that a familial factor – or factors – strongly influences later sexual behavior. The more recent twin studies of homosexuality grew directly out of earlier ones that repeatedly confirmed an unequivocal family influence. In its 1973 decision that homosexuality was not an illness, the American Psychological Association ignored almost eighty years' worth of psychoanalytic and psychotherapeutic observation. The gist of these practitioners' observations is consistent with what more rigorous scientific data demonstrates, namely, that the family environment plays a critical role in the development of homosexuality.

What did the psychoanalysts learn that activists want us to forget? That in the lives of their homosexual patients there was unusually often an emotional mismatch between the child and same-sex parent (such as a father who subtly or overtly rejects a son who has many "feminine" traits); or an emotional mismatch between the child and the opposite sex parent; or sexual abuse of a child by either the same sex or opposite sex parent; and most often the rejection of a child by same-sex peers.

Many excellent psychoanalytic and psychotherapeutic studies describe the complex interactions among these and other factors. Although these studies do not identify or describe any innate components that influence these environmental factors, they generate likely hypotheses to be further tested about the environmental influences on homosexuality evident in the genetics research.

Besides the influence of the family, various other theories of homosexuality have evolved out of the extensive clinical experience of psychoanalysts and psychotherapists. It is not my purpose to provide or critique a detailed survey of these various theories; rather, my scientific purpose is served by demonstrating that the question regarding the precise causes of homosexuality remains open.

Nonetheless, we will look at what might be termed a "soft" consensus that has emerged over the years within the clinical community about how homosexuality occurs and changes. This consensus concerns a number of developmental events and sequences that lead to the habitual use of anxiety-reducing, self-soothing behaviors, including sexual deviations, promiscuity, homosexuality, and many other activities. Quite often an individual will use more than one such outlet. Thus, for example, homosexuality is commonly associated with both promiscuity and alcoholism or drug use. These activities all have a transiently soothing effect and the tendency to become first habitual, then compulsive, and finally addictive.

The developmental events and sequences that give rise to these later problems, though different from case to case, nonetheless share certain general features. These may be lumped together under the heading "psychic trauma."

"Psychic trauma" is a subtle concept that needs explaining. For one thing, actual physical trauma, including sexual abuse, may well be the source of psychic trauma. In the specific case of homosexuality it often appears to be the source. Nonetheless, actual physical trauma does not have to occur to cause psychic trauma. Also, individuals differ in their innate susceptibility to be traumatized. A severe, life-changing trauma for one individual may have little effect in another; conversely, what most outside observers rate as a trivial event could seriously wound someone with a particular disposition.

And so when we think of 'trauma' we are apt to conceptualize it *objectively*, as a measurable outer event. This kind of trauma lends itself to quantitative research. One example is the studies that have found a disproportionate extent of sexual abuse in the childhoods of adult homosexuals.

But psychic trauma is actually a purely subjective experience. The link between psychic trauma and measurable external influences can vary from tight and obvious to loose and invisible. Parental behavior, for example, can range from being, as many unprejudiced observers would agree, "bad" to being "good," while still being poorly matched to the needs of the child through no fault of the parent.

Thus inner-oriented approaches to the concept of "psychic trauma" or "wounding" – whether secular (meaning psychoanalytic) or spiritual – provide a necessary additional perspective. For practical reasons, however, this perspective will remain almost invisible to rigorous scientific methods.

The kinds of traumas that can result in disturbed behavior are many and varied. Two specific traumas are most commonly associated with homosexuality.

The first is the trauma caused by the child's subjective experience of the same-sex parent's lack of availability, rejection, or even harsh verbal, physical, or sexual attack. By objective standards, the parent himself or herself may or may not be described in these terms. Rather the child's subjective experience of the parent creates the effect. This may give rise to the child's profound longing for love from that parent, a longing that he or she will likely enact in later relations with peers of the same sex. This longing may also become sexualized, that is, linked to the distress-relieving capacity of orgasm.

The results of a study by George Rekers reflect this:

> Significantly fewer male role models were found
> in the family backgrounds of the severely gender-dis-

turbed boys as compared to the mild-to-moderately gender-disturbed boys. Male childhood gender disturbance was also found to be correlated with a high incidence of psychiatric problems in both the mothers and fathers and with atypical patterns of the boys' involvement with their mothers and fathers. . . .

The second is the trauma caused by the child's subjective experience of the opposite-sex parent's lack of availability, rejection, or even harsh verbal, physical, or sexual attack. This may give rise to the child's fear of that parent, which will likely show itself later as a heightened wariness and avoidance of opposite-sex relations.

We must add a caution, however. Although these kinds of trauma are unusually common in the childhoods of homosexuals, they are not universal. And in many cases other, less typical traumas *are* present. This reflects the inherent complexity of homosexuality, a complexity stemming from the interactive or multiple genetic, intrauterine, environmental, family, social, psychological, and habitual influences on the course of development. Thus even common, quite general disturbances in family life, such as parental separation, are associated with a measurably increased incidence of homosexuality. Such general disturbances are more readily quantified than the inner experience of psychic trauma.

Other possible causes of psychic trauma abound; the literature is filled with case studies that show many different kinds of childhood backgrounds. This diversity of experience does not mean that *all* possible childhood experiences lead to homosexuality and therefore that none do. It reflects, rather, that the *compulsive pursuit of pleasure (of all sorts) is the most common human response to distress.*

Conclusion

Ours is not the first era to embrace, for social and political reason, a biological theory of homosexuality. The idea was first floated in the late 1800s, especially in England and on the continent but foundered quickly as soon as people began to look more closely. The 1890s forgotten, the notion became a genuine fad in Germany of the 1930s, once again without evidence. The 1930s forgotten – at

Jeffrey Satinover

least that aspect – the theory has risen once again, this time not only once again with no evidence, but with more solid evidence *against* it.

The Gay Deception
Joseph Nicolosi, Ph.D.

I would like to consider in this chapter the process by which someone comes to define or identify himself as "gay." My view is based upon the clinical treatment of over 400 homosexually oriented men during eighteen years as a practicing psychologist. My view is that "gay" is a self-deceptive identity. This "gay" identity has been brilliantly marketed by a small number of people who are consciously pursuing an agenda. It has been accepted, often uncritically, by many within the most influential institutions of American society – professional psychology and psychiatry, churches, education, and the media.

"Gay" Is Not "Homosexual"

It is important to distinguish between someone who is "homosexual" and someone who is "gay." A "homosexual" is anyone who experiences a sexual attraction to persons of the same sex. Only some "homosexuals" are "gay." "Homosexuals" who regard their attraction as disordered are not "gay" and do not describe themselves as "gay." The man who recognizes that he has a homosexual problem and struggles to overcome it is, simply, "homosexual."

"Gay" is a self identity chosen by some homosexuals. The gay-identified person identifies himself with the idea that homosexual behavior is as normal and natural as heterosexual behavior. "Gays" are therefore homosexuals who morally approve of same-sex sexual activity, and regard their own participation in such activity as normal and desirable.

What, then, do I mean when I say that "gay" is a self-deceptive identity? I mean that "gay" is a fictitious identity seized upon by

Joseph Nicolosi, Ph. D.

an individual to resolve painful emotional challenges. "Gay" – which is to say, self-identification as "gay" – is an often sincere, but always misguided, attempt to cope with real problems, albeit tragically, by denying significant aspects of human reality. "Gay" is an escape, one which often begins in childhood.

Development of a "gay" identity takes place through three basic steps in a psycho-social process. It begins, first, with the pre-homosexual child and his gender distortions, followed by his later assimilation into the "gay" counterculture, which fosters those same distortions about self and about life. The final step involves the "gay" community's expansion of its self-deception into the further deception of a large portion of society.

Early Gender Identity

At a critical developmental period called the gender-identity phase, the young child discovers that the world is divided between male and female. The child is challenged to assume male-ness or femaleness. "Am I a boy? Or am I a girl?"

Confronted with the reality of a gendered world, male and female, and forced to make a choice, the child may first resort to an avoidance strategy – regressing into an androgynous phase: "I need not relinquish the benefits of either sex. I can be both male and female." In psychoanalytic terms, he can have a penis and make babies. However, reality pushes in and language now enters, and he hears "he" and "she," and "his" and "hers."

Both boys and girls are first identified with the mother, their "first love object" – but the boy has the additional developmental task of disentangling his identity from his mother and identifying with the father. (We will be talking primarily about boys here, because male homosexuality is the predominant and more cultur-ally aggressive form in our society, and because there are some sig-nificant developmental differences along the path to lesbianism.) Make no mistake about this: masculinity, as Robert Stoller said, is an *achievement*. The child – especially the boy – has to work not only for the acquisition of identity, but for the acquisition of gen-der. Every culture that has ever survived understands this matter of the achievement of gender, and will support and assist the boy through rites of passage and male initiation.

Today we are rapidly abandoning support of our sons' formation of masculine identity, especially the support essential to that formation which comes from parents. The father is the most significant person in the identification process. If the father is warm and receptive and inviting, the boy will not identify with the mother. He will instead bond with the father to fulfill his natural masculine strivings. If the father is cold, detached, harsh, or simply disinterested, the boy *may* reach out to his father. But, eventually, he will feel hurt and discouraged, and surrender his natural masculine strivings. Then he will return to his mother.

While there is no convincing scientific evidence of a "gay gene," certain boys do seem especially vulnerable to homosexual development. Clinical experience tells us that the boy who is sensitive, passive, gentle, and aesthetically oriented may be most susceptible to retreat from the developmental challenge to gender-identify with his father. A tougher, bolder, thicker-skinned son may well succeed in pushing through an emotional barrier. But the sensitive son thinks, "I can't be male, but I'm not completely female either; so I will remain in my own little androgynous world, my secret place of fantasy."

This quality of androgynous fantasy is a fundamental feature of gay culture. This fantasy contains within it, not only the narcissistic refusal to identify with a gendered culture, but also the refusal to identify with the human biological reality upon which our gendered society is based. In fact, gender – a core feature of personal identity – is central to the way we relate to ourselves and others. It is also a central pathway through which we grow to maturity.

A host of studies confirm the correlation between childhood gender nonconformity, which is suggestive of gender-identity confusion, and later homosexuality. Not all homosexuality develops this way, but this is a common developmental pathway. We hear echoes of this theme over and over in gay literature – the repeated story of the pre-homosexual boy who is isolated and "on the outs" from male friends, feeling different, insecure in his male-ness and alone, disenfranchised from father, and retreating back to mother.

Because gender was such a source of pain in childhood, the annihilation of gender differences is, not surprisingly, a central theme of gay culture. Gays often call their attitude "an indiffer-ence to gender." One well-known theorist, himself a gay man, spoke recently of his own utopian society as a "non-gender-polar-izing culture" in which everyone would potentially be anyone else's lover.

Detachment from Self and Others

The person who accepts the gay label in adulthood has typi-cally spent much of his childhood emotionally disconnected from people, particularly his male peers and his father. He also was likely to assume a false, rigid "good little boy" role within the fam-ily.

One of my clients said, "I was a non-entity. I didn't have a place to feel like myself." Another man said, "I always acted out other people's scripts for me. I was an actor in other people's plays." Still another client reported, "My parents watched me grow up." Upon hearing this, another man added, "I watched myself grow up." That quality of detachment from self is evident in all these assertions, and they are typical of reports from my clientele as a whole. No wonder the pre-homosexual boy is often interested in theatre and acting. Life is theatre. We are all actors. Reality is what we wish it to be.

This detachment hinders development of an authentic identi-ty, one grounded in healthy adjustments to the realities of gender acquisition. The pre-homosexual boy then begins to enter the "gay" world by re-inventing himself. Oscar Wilde (who probably was the first person to give a face to "gay"), said, "Naturalness is just another pose." Without domestic emotional bonds to ground him in organic identity, the man is plastic. He is the transformist, a Victor-Victoria, or the character from "La Cage Aux Folles." He is a pretender, a jokester – what French psychoanalyst Chasseguet-Smirge calls "the imposter."

Freud said, "The father is the reality principle." Father represents the transition from the blissful mother-child relationship into harsh reality. But the pre-homosexual boy says to himself, "If my father makes me unimportant, I make him unimportant. If he rejects me, I reject him and all that he represents." The boy says: "Father has nothing to teach me. His power to procreate and affect the world are nothing compared to my fantasy world. What he accomplishes, I can dream. Dream and reality are the same."

Rather than striving to find his own masculine, procreative power and moving out into the world, the pre-homosexual boy chooses instead to stay in a dream-filled world of his own imagining. He has a sense of not being a part of other people's lives, and begins to exhibit that narcissism and preoccupation with self – traits commonly observed in male homosexuals. The pre-homosexual boy is detached, not only from father and other boys, but from maleness and his own male body, including the first symbol of masculinity, his own penis – an object alien even to himself. Homosexual behavior is the search for the lost masculine self.

By the early teenage years, unconscious drives to fill this emotional vacuum – to want to connect with his maleness – are felt as homoerotic desires. The next stage will be entry into the gay world. Then for the first time in his life, this lonely, alienated young man meets (through gay romance novels from the library, TV personalities, or Internet chat rooms, for example) people who share the same feelings. But he gets more than empathy: along with the empathy comes an entire package of new ideas and concepts about sex, gender, human relationships, anatomical relationships, and personal destiny.

Next he experiences that heady, euphoric, rite-of-passage called "coming out of the closet." It is just one more constructed role to distract him from the deeper, more painful issue of self-identity. "Gay" identity is thus not "discovered," as if it existed *a priori* as a natural trait. It is, rather, a culturally approved process of self-reinvention by a group of people in order to mask their collective emotional hurts. This claim to have finally found authentic identity through gayness is perhaps the most perilous of all the false roles attempted by the young person seeking identity and belonging. One of the benefits of membership in the gay sub-culture is the support and reinforcement he receives for reverting to fantasy as a method of problem solving.

What awesome benefits the young man receives by assuming the "gay" self-label! Potentially unlimited sex. Vast power or mastery over others and his environment. Why? Because the retreat into group fantasy, bringing with it a sense of belonging to an outlaw culture, frees the young "gay" man from feelings of inadequacy and loneliness that permeated his life in "straight" culture. A world not to his liking is eliminated from consciousness, replaced by a world called into being precisely to validate the "gay" resolution of his problems. He also enjoys vindication of early childhood hurts and, as an added bonus, he gets to reject his rejecting father.

The "Gay" Cosmic Make Over

How has this group of hurt boys and girls – now known in adulthood as the "gay" community – managed to promote their make-believe liberation, not only to popular culture but to legislators, public-policy makers, universities, and churches?

There are a number of ways and explanations. Four deserve special mention.

The first is the "gay" community's appropriation of the rhetoric of the civil-rights movement, probably the single most influential force in forming the collective consciousness of American society in this century. Gay apologists have exploited authentic rights issues as a wedge to promote their redefinition of human sexuality and, essentially, human nature. (I say "authentic rights issues" because, as the Catholic Church teaches, all persons, including the self-deceiving gay person, have the same human rights. Irrational hostility to such persons has, indeed, sometimes led to denial of their rights.)

One powerful rhetorical tool used time and time again by "gays" is what I call "The Coming Out Story." It is that same generic story that has been repeated almost verbatim for thirty years now, from the committee rooms of the American Psychiatric Association in 1973 to the Oprah Winfrey Show. "Finding oneself" and "being who one really is" are popular late-twentieth-century themes which have a heroic and attractive ring to them. Certainly the person telling the story is sincere. He means what he says, but the audience rarely looks beyond his words to understand his "coming out" in the larger context.

A second factor is that sexuality itself is in crisis, with fundamental changes now taking place in our definition of family, community, procreation, marriage, and gender. All of these changes have occurred in the interest of the individual right to pursue sexual pleasure. The gay movement historically followed along on the coattails of the civil-rights movement and adopted much of its rhetoric. It also draws ideological power from the sexual-liberation movement.

A third explanation for the "gay" movement's successful move toward the mainstream of our society is commercial. Ours is a consumer-oriented society, and consumer products shape our view of ourselves. Marketing strategists are all-too-ready to target consumer groups. Gay couples are called "DINKS" – dual income, no kids. And that means expendable income. Merchants have always been ready to cater to gay clientele, and merchant-solicitors have given the gay community the face of legitimacy. Today, nearly every major corporation offers services specially tailored to homosexuals – corporations like AT&T, Hyatt House, Seagrams, Apple Computer, Time-Warner, and American Express. Alcohol and cigarettes are popular gay items. We see gay resorts, gay cruises, gay theatre, gay film festivals, gay magazines, movies, and fiction give face and theme to individuals whose essential problems are identity and belonging. Luxury items such as jewelry, fashion, furnishings, and cosmetics are ready to soothe, flatter, and gratify a hurting minority. But beyond material reassurance, these luxury items equate gay identity with economic success: "the gay life is the good life."

Finally, the "gay" movement is easily rationalized by the arguments of deconstructionism, probably the most fashionable ideology on the American college scene. The founder of the deconstructionist movement is Michel Foucault, a "gay" whose philosophical views emerged out of his own personal struggle with homosexuality. Foucault actually had the outrageous plan to deconstruct the distinction between life and death; in his later years, he was obsessed with the idea of simultaneously experiencing death and orgasm. He eventually succeeded at least in deconstructing himself. (Foucault died of AIDS in a sanitarium.)

Deconstructionism and the gay agenda are perfectly compatible. They both subsist on the upending of traditional distinctions and the obliteration of differences grounded in nature – that is, metaphysics. And so through deconstructionism we see animal confused with human, sacred confused with profane, adult confused with child, male confused with female, and life confused with death – all of these, traditionally the most profound of distinctions and separations, are now under siege through modern deconstructionism.

The Way Out

And so we have seen that gay is a compromise identity seized upon by an individual, and increasingly supported by our society, in order to resolve emotional conflicts. It is a collective illusion; truly, "the gay deception." But I have seen more men than I can count in the process of struggle, growth and change. The struggle is a soul-searing one, as it must be, for it challenges an identity rooted in one's earliest years.

As adults, these strugglers have looked into the gay lifestyle and return disillusioned by what they saw. Rather than wage war against the natural order of society, they have chosen to take up the challenge of an interior struggle. This is, I am convinced, the only true existential solution to an age-old identity problem.

Does Homosexuality Nullify a Marriage?
Canon Law and Recent Developments in Psychology and Psychiatry*
Monsignor Cormac Burke

Can a person with a homosexual tendency validly consent to marriage? In this chapter I shall recall established principles of canon law, and apply them to the case of homosexuality, taking into account recent changes in psychological and psychiatric evaluations of homosexuality. We shall examine these changes and weigh their possible effect on canonical jurisprudence. These changes are not, as is so often stated, strictly scientific or "value free," and must be critically evaluated in light of a proper Christian anthropology.

I
Principles of Morality and Canon Law

Canonical jurisprudence, as articulated in the authoritative judgments of the Roman Rota (the Vatican tribunal in charge of marriage and annulment cases), holds that homosexuality "is a disorder of the instinct or that natural tendency (psychologically, physically and effectively) of one sex towards the other, which in the nature of things...leads and urges people to that union of man and woman which is marriage."[1] Homosexuality is considered a "pathological state of the sexual instinct."[2]

It is likewise established that incapacity for assuming certain matrimonial obligations "occurs in some grave cases of homosexuality." These cases "can certainly not be harmonized with the nature of matrimonial consent."[3] In other words, not every expression of homosexuality impedes matrimonial consent. "Homosexuality can only do so when one or other spouse suffers from true, i.e. *grave and irreversible* homosexuality."[4] (Emphasis added.)

Canonical jurisprudence distinguishes not only between grave and less grave cases of homosexuality, but also between a homosexual tendency that is transient and one that is deep-rooted, and again between an acquired homosexual condition and one that would seem to be constitutional. "Among those who suffer a perversion or rather an inversion in the erotic appetite, one needs to distinguish those who give way to this aberration only transiently and on certain occasions, or impelled by circumstances of place or time, and who easily return to the right order when freed from these circumstances; these without doubt are in a totally different situation to others who either out of a habit firmly contracted over a long period (i.e. who have become homosexuals), or from their own constitutional makeup (who are therefore abnormal from birth), are irresistibly attracted to their own sex which medical opinion considers to have originated in an organic cause or from a pathological psychic condition."[5]

In relation to the proof of an incapacitating homosexual condition, "there must be proof of the gravity and the incurability of the [homosexual] disorder. For a slight inhibition or one that can be cured would give rise to an imperfect and perhaps also unhappy marriage, over a period or indefinitely. But the object of an incapacity is a null marriage, not one that is simply imperfect or difficult to live up to."[6]

II
Recent Developments in Psychology and Psychiatry

The question could be asked: to what extent should these received principles of rotal decisionmaking be modified, in light of the radically changed position of so much of the secular world with regard to homosexuality?

Until twenty or thirty years ago, homosexual conduct, even between consenting adults, was treated as a criminal offense in civil law, and was socially considered an unacceptable deviation. This was reflected in psychiatry, where it was universally held to be a psychic illness needing therapeutic attention. In 1973, however, the American Psychiatric Association (more specifically, its board), eliminated the classification of homosexuality as a mental disorder. In 1980 the APA restricted any diagnosis of pathology to cases where homosexuality caused subjective distress, so-called "ego-dystonic" homosexuality. The APA limited this further in 1987, and in 1994 finally removed homosexuality completely from any categorization as a personality disorder. These developments found expression in successive editions of the *Diagnostic and Statistical Manual of Mental Disorders* (DSM), put out by the APA itself.

The development of psychiatric thinking about homosexuality, as expressed in the successive editions of the DSM, has had wide and deep effects. The DSM is not only utilized by the American psychiatric profession, but has now become a manual of international use, having been translated into all the leading languages. The importance of this for jurisprudential purposes is all the more evident when one recalls that, in cases concerning possible consensual incapacity for marriage, canonical tribunals have come to rely heavily on experts in psychiatry and psychology, while these experts themselves tend to invoke DSM more and more. Judges tend to have a copy of DSM to hand and very frequently ask experts to give their diagnoses using DSM classifications, in the conviction that this provides the judge with a means to calibrate the scientific reliability of an expert opinion. In rotal jurisprudence, DSM is described as a "renowned work," "easily the leading account of mental disorders," "the greatly used text," "the constantly used list of mental disorders," and its terminology as the "commonly recognized listing." In rotal sentences of the period 1990–1995 which treat of consensual incapacity, DSM is referred to some 200 times.

Given this extensive reliance upon DSM, two main questions about it urgently call for consideration: (1) its reliability, from the strictly scientific viewpoint, as a trustworthy source of unbiased knowledge; (2) its harmony with the Christian concept of man. To these two questions I now turn.

III
The Hidden Values of the Therapeutic Sciences

There is considerable professional disagreement among psychiatrists themselves about whether the development of DSM has always been shaped by purely scientific judgments.

Doubts about the scientific objectivity of the DSM were widely aired within the psychiatric profession after the publication of DSM-III, in 1980. Dr. Alan A. Stone, Professor of Law and Psychiatry at Harvard University and 1980 President of the American Psychiatric Association, observed: "One of the first great battlefields in the attack on psychiatry's hidden values was homosexuality. Psychiatrists had long assumed that as part of their humanistic tradition they had brought their scientific perspective to things that were once considered evil. Homosexuality became sickness rather than sin, and this perspective in this century was accepted not only by the secular masses but even by most religious authorities. However, gay liberation brought a different perspective. Their argument was that our judgments about homosexuality as sickness contained hidden values, a limited vision of human sensuality and intimacy, the old morality under a new guise, and perhaps even our own phobic limitations. A campaign was undertaken to remove the diagnosis of homosexuality from the nomenclature. Our Association, after considerable deliberation and not a little acrimony, accepted that perspective. Our Association went even further – it called for an end to legal discrimination against homosexuality."[7]

The *American Journal of Psychiatry* in 1984 carried an important "Debate on DSM-III" with Dr. Robert L. Spitzer, Professor of Psychiatry at Columbia University, New York, and the main mind behind DSM-III, responding to criticisms from other prominent psychiatrists. This debate shows that even supporters of DSM-III admit the unscientific character of many of the changes it introduces, and urge that future developments should be more solidly based.

These self-doubts about the reliability of DSM continue to be voiced at the highest level within the psychiatric profession. In a recent editorial of the *American Journal of Psychiatry*, we read: "the new DSM diagnostic process has dominated the research, teaching, and contemporary practice of psychiatry... The DSM diagnosis has become the main goal of clinical practice. DSM-IV, as 'allegedly' being more data-based, has even assumed the aura of allowing psychiatry to keep pace with the rest of medicine as a 'technological triumph';... all of this apparent precision overlooks the fact that as yet, we have no identified etiological agents for psychiatric disorders. Our diagnoses are nowhere near the precision of the diagnostic processes in the rest of medicine."[8]

IV
Evaluating the Hidden Biases

What can we make of these misgivings, voiced by leaders within the psychiatric profession itself, about the non-scientific influences upon the DSM and its treatment of homosexuality ? How much science – and how much bias – is there in the DSM?

Few psychiatrists would deny that concepts of "psychic health" are enormously influenced by prevailing norms of personal or social behavior, giving rise to the danger that both psychiatry and psychology can be subordinated to, or manipulated by, prevailing cultural or class values. This danger has often been noted in the past, and it is certainly not less operative today. We quote from an article by Dr. J. Eaton: "Cultural relativity plays a much larger role in the fields of mental health and illness than in most other fields of medicine. An inflamed appendix has a fairly uniform meaning in all cultures that recognize life as a desirable value. If left untreated it is a threat to life. Not so in the mental field. Even in the case of very unusual behavior, like suicide, one cannot find complete cross-cultural uniformity in its interpretation. . . . [I]n the United States the mental hygiene movement has accepted the democratic, worldly ascetic, individualistic, utilitarian, and competitive values of the middle class. Its criteria for mental health reflects strong personal and class biases and are in part rejected by other sections of the population."[9]

Eaton emphasizes that "[p]sychiatrists and clinical psychologists have personal criteria of the requirements to consider a patient cured. These criteria arise out of their experiences and social value orientation. No common denominator for these definitions can be found."[10] Eaton also observes: "Afrank recognition of the relativity of mental health will do much to improve both research and its application. It will reduce confusion by putting an end to the fruitless effort to arrive at a single criterion, which some scientists hope would be endowed through some magical process with the "objectivity" of temperature measured by a thermometer. Mental health cannot be reduced to such a single dimension. It is a value judgment, with all the potentialities for variation and change implicit in such a relativistic entity."[11]

In dealing with the troubled workings of the human spirit, psychiatry inevitably (even if, perhaps, unconsciously in some cases) adopts a series of philosophically or morally based *value judgments* about "concepts of self," about man himself, his nature, his development and end, his psychic good and health.

It is significant to find opinions from such authoritative voices within the psychiatric profession, insisting that theirs is not an exact science, but one which relies heavily on "value judgments," on philosophy and anthropology, and also on theses rooted in sociological premises. A recent article in the *British Journal of Psychiatry* (which holds that psychiatry "is a social practice") stresses "the new approach to psychiatric knowledge which is developed under the influence of social anthropology over the last decade," and asserts that psychiatry "is too socially embedded in the sense that it cannot examine its own institutional assumptions, and mistakes the particular for the universal."[12]

V

A Christian View of Man and Scientific Opinions in Marriage Cases

Reflecting on all of the above, the canonist's mind is naturally drawn to the 1987 Address of Pope John Paul II to the Roman Rota. There the Pope insisted on the ecclesiastical judge's responsibility, in marriage nullity cases, to detect and evaluate the anthropological or philosophical presuppositions that necessarily underlie a psychiatric or psychological opinion. The Holy Father warned of the "the very grave danger . . . as regards decisions about the nullity of marriages" if the judge, unaware that "the anthropological view, which underpins so many currents of thought in the field of modern psychological science is as a whole irreconcilable with the essential elements of Christian anthropology," were to give judicial weight to expertise based on false anthropological presuppositions.[13]

Even if the majority of psychiatrists – for whatever reasons – were to conclude that homosexuality is no longer to be considered a disorder, Christian anthropology cannot accept this conclusion. According to the Christian understanding of man, human nature, weakened though not intrinsically corrupted by Original Sin, is beset in almost all of its faculties and powers by disordered tendencies, whose presence there calls for a constant struggle. Every normal person experiences these disturbed tendencies in a particularly strong way in the whole area of sexuality. Hence the concept of "normality," in regard even to heterosexuality, is somewhat equivocal, for the "normal" *hetero*sexual person also experiences disorders and must continuously strive to correct or check these deviations, so as to keep his or her balance in what is a basically turbulent situation.

The *Catechism of the Catholic Church*, treating of sexuality in general, insists that it needs proper integration into the existence of each person – a vital task that cannot be achieved without the exercise of the virtue of chastity and the use of human and supernatural means. "All the baptized are called to chastity [which] means the successful integration of sexuality within the person"; "Chastity includes an apprenticeship in self-mastery which is a training in human freedom. The alternative is clear: either man governs his passions and finds peace, or he lets himself be dominated by them and becomes unhappy"; "Self-mastery is a long and exacting work. One can never consider it acquired once and for all. It presupposes renewed effort at all stages of life."[14]

On this background, the *Catechism* goes on to speak of homosexuality. "Homosexuality refers to relations between men or between women who experience an exclusive or predominant sexual attraction toward persons of the same sex. Tradition has always declared that homosexual acts are intrinsically disordered. They are contrary to the natural law. . . . Under no circumstances can they be approved. . . . The number of men and women who have deep-seated homosexual tendencies is not negligible. They do not choose their homosexual condition; for most of them it is a trial. . . . These persons are called to fulfil God's will in their lives and, if they are Christians, to unite to the sacrifice of the Lord's Cross the difficulties they may encounter from their condition. . . . Homosexual persons are called to chastity. By the virtues of self-mastery that teach them inner freedom. . . by prayer and sacramental grace, they can and should gradually and resolutely approach Christian perfection."[15]

The Church therefore holds that homosexuality is a disorder, whether considered as inclination or as conduct. It naturally distinguishes between homosexual tendency, which in itself has nothing sinful to it, and homosexual practice which is always sinful – just as it distinguishes between the strong but not-consented-to temptation to infidelity in a married person, and actual adultery on that person's part. The insistence on the possession and application of Christian anthropological standards calls on courts, as well as court experts, to check on their own working presuppositions. If a judge lacks a due grasp of Christian anthropology, he is likely to uncritically absorb the operative values underlying each expertise, and be unable to fulfill his mission of deciding whether or not they are acceptable and applicable from a Christian point of view. Not all experts whose services are regularly used by tribunals seem to be as aware of the fact that while most of secular psychology considers certain dispositions or practices to be mutually incompatible or exclusive, Christian thought sees them as complementary and intrinsically designed for integration: freedom and commitment; self-fulfillment and self-denial; "autotomy" and "relatedness"; maturity and dependence. Secular psychologists quite regularly see "over-dependence" or "over-acceptance" as signs of an immature personality. A Catholic would be extremely cautious about applying such a criterion, above all when it comes to judging capacity for marriage which, in a Christian understanding, is a way of life that calls for a high degree of both mutual acceptance and mutual dependence.

The relationship between frequently invoked psychological concepts, such as "self-esteem" and "freedom from shame or guilt," or "self-doubt" and "self-actualization," would probably be interpreted quite differently according to whether one has a Christian or a secularist anthropological outlook. The same would hold, no doubt, for the nature and psychological evaluation of "self-image" or "self-assertion," or for the concepts of "validation" or of "healing."

The idea that people can be in "syntony" – in positive emotional response – with a bad or unworthy tendency is a logical consequence of the current philosophy of "self-definition," which opposes the notion of a given human nature, common to all, and therefore cannot accept that certain actions are "natural" and others "anti-natural." It holds that each person rather has the absolute right to define oneself, one's goals, and the parameters of personal conduct which one considers "acceptable," all of which undoubtedly facilitates the ego-syntonic goal of "being at peace with oneself." In this view, conscience loses its character as a higher, independent, and critical voice of truth and is reduced to an ego-syntonically regulated stamp of approval placed by the subject on whatever he or she wants to do.

The Church has always rejected this total moral subjectivism, this self-threatening current of thought in which freedom is exalted "to such an extent that it becomes an absolute, which would then be the source of values . . . in this way the inescapable claims of truth disappear, yielding their place to a criterion of sincerity, authenticity and 'being at peace with oneself'. . ."[16]

Even if morality is left aside, two questions can be posed from the purely psychological point of view. First, is it possible that a person can feel "ego-syntonic" – that is, completely "at peace" and experiencing no personal distress at all – about any action or form of conduct whatsoever that he or she claims to consider acceptable: murder or rape for instance? Secondly, if one allows that this is possible, can such subjective tranquility about objectively inhuman conduct be taken as a sign of psychic normality, or ought it rather not be considered proof of grave mental pathology?

VI

The Canon Law of Marriage and Homosexuality

As a possible canonical ground of the nullity of marriage, homosexuality is treated almost exclusively within the ambit of canon (abbreviated hereafter as "c.") 1095. C. 1095 refers to "a grave defect of discretion" – or incapacity – which undermines the apparent consent to the marriage." This should not be permitted to lead to a neglect of its possible relevance under the terms of c. 1098. If, in order to bring about marital consent a person deliberately conceals a deep-rooted homosexual tendency, a *prima facie* cast is already present for a declaration of nullity, since such a condition certainly "of its very nature can seriously disturb the partnership of conjugal life" (cf. c. 1098). If what had been deliberately concealed were not just a homosexual tendency, but previous homosexual activity, the case would be so much stronger.

As we saw from the principles enunciated earlier, jurisprudence is agreed that a grave homosexual condition, present at consent, can provoke consensual incapacity under c. 1095(3). Care must be taken however lest judgments in this field be too absolute. Otherwise there is the danger of converting certain psychic anomalies which provoke consensual incapacity in *particular* circumstances (when the anomaly is grave; when the married obligations for which it incapacitates are constitutionally essential) into matrimonial impediments in *all* circumstances – which is clearly not the legislator's intent as expressed in c. 1095.

No small number of cases coming to the Rota suggest that for some judges and experts, the slightest evidence that some of the diagnostic criteria proposed by DSM for identifying a psychic disorder were present at the time of consent suffices to *prove* a party's incapacity for marriage under c. 1095. Such a practice ignores two evident facts: (1) DSM in its explicit desire to be exhaustive, classifies many "disorders" which cannot be even remotely connected with capacity for the *essential obligations of marriage* (as c. 1095 requires); (2) no less importantly, it passes over the clear principle, long established in rotal jurisprudence and recalled in 1987 by Pope John Paul II that "an argument for real incapacity can be entertained only in the presence of a serious form of anomaly . . .."[17] The editors of DSM-IV seem to have wished to preclude such superficial reading or use of their manual when they write in their introduction: "It is precisely because impairments, abilities, and disabilities vary widely within each diagnostic category that assignment of a particular diagnosis does not imply a specific level of impairment or disability."[18]

The editors add another "caveat" which is specially significant for those who habitually have recourse to DSM for canonical cases under c. 1095. "The fact that an individual's presentation meets the criteria for a DSM-IV diagnosis does not carry any necessary implication regarding the individual's degree of control over the behaviors that may be associated with the disorder. Even when diminished control over one's behavior is a feature of the disorder, having the diagnosis in itself does not demonstrate that a particular individual is (or was) unable to control his or her behavior at a particular time."[19] This distinction in DSM between "diminished control" and "inability to control" corresponds to the distinction in canonical jurisprudence between "difficulty" – which does not invalidate consent – and "incapacity," which does. This is firmly established in rotal jurisprudence, and was also recalled by the Pope in his address to the Rota in 1997: "For the canonist the principle is clear that *incapacity* alone, and not just *difficulty*, in giving consent and achieving a true community of life and love, renders marriage null."[20]

This caution applies to other conditions that are frequently dealt with under c. 1095. A formal sentence of consensual incapacity not only takes away the ecclesial right to marry of the person so judged, but deprives anyone wishing to marry him or her of the same right at least as regards the marriage desired. No one can marry a person incapable of valid marriage consent. While the point may have less importance in regard to no. 2 of c. 1095 (a "grave defect of discretion" can at times be of a transitory nature), it calls for attentive consideration with respect to certain chronic or constitutional conditions that are at times invoked as grounds for the "incapacity of assuming" of no. 3 of the canon.

Declarations of nullity which correspond to truth and justice serve to protect and uphold ecclesial rights. Such rights, however, can be undermined if the principles underlying a declaration of nullity are not properly grounded in justice. It is only for very grave and solidly proven reasons that a person can be deprived of the natural and ecclesial right to marry (cf. c. 1058).

According to established jurisprudence, as we have noted, a mild or moderate homosexual condition does not justify a declaration of consensual incapacity. Several reasons bear out the prudence of this.

1. A "real" homosexual has an exclusive sexual attraction toward persons of the same sex and, at the same time, not simply a mere lack of such attraction but an actual *repugnance* regarding physical sexual relations with persons of the opposite sex. "When faced with a homosexual subject a first question of major importance must always be made: that is, whether it is a case of a constitutional homosexual or of one that should be considered 'occasional.' To be justified in speaking of a real homosexual, i.e. of one who is constitutionally so, it is not enough that there be an attraction towards persons of the same sex. It is necessary that there also be a distaste for the other sex. Every homosexual who does not fulfil this last condition is probably an occasional homosexual. . . . The true homosexual is an instinctual deviant in the proper sense of the term: everything occurs in him as if he were born of an element carrying sexual inversion in itself."[21]

2. To have (or to have had, in the past) a *certain* homosexual tendency is by no means infrequent. Whether persons with such a tendency are properly classified under the heading of "bisexual" (having a sexual orientation toward people of either sex) is a question that may be of interest to the psychiatrist, but it is not important to the ecclesiastical judge, since it is clear that such persons cannot be barred from exercising the right to marry. Their natural attraction to marriage remains and, if they marry, their usual motive is love for their partner. A recent study in a psychological review makes this point (in relation to lesbians): "The great major-

ity of bisexual or lesbian women reported that they got married because they were in love with their husbands and desired marriage . . . studies indicate that their marriages may be no more conflicted than heterosexual marriages."[22]

3. The sentence of one appeals court seemed to look positively on the contention that one can "speak of a homosexual tendency of antecedent gravity, and for this very reason incompatible with the assumption of matrimonial life." Here there is the danger of failing to distinguish, not only between tendency and practice, but also between a bad tendency, which simply reflects fallen nature, and the curbing of that tendency which, along with showing moral strength, can also be inspired by love for one's partner.

There can be no grounds for holding that an immoral tendency, *if resisted*, can incapacitate a person for the undertaking or fulfillment of any essential marital obligation. Otherwise it would follow that someone highly subject to sexual temptation is incapable of validly marrying, since he or she will go through married life with a constant urge to infidelity – although he is also determined to resist those temptations and has hitherto normally succeeded in doing so. This is surely not correct. Moreover, even if occasional falls were to occur during actual married life, it would seem impossible to conclude with certainty that this was due to incapacity, and not just to difficulty.

A tendency cannot be held to cause incapacity. We all have tendencies to act perversely. For the juridic proof of consensual incapacity, what has to be established is not the anomaly or pathology of having wrong tendencies, nor even that of yielding to them (which per se simply shows a *voluntary* giving way to a bad moral inclination), but the anomaly of *not being capable of* resisting them.

Nor is this clear principle undermined by an expert opinion to the effect that the tendency in question is "constitutional" or "inherited." If the tendency is held in check, so that a person's *con-duct* remains within the norm, the tendency cannot incapacitate. It is not a tendency which one manages to control, but conduct which one cannot control, that can sustain an allegation of incapacity under c. 1095(3).

4. The mutual exchange of the right to true conjugal acts is essential to the constitution of marriage. According to c. 1084(1), impotence or the inability to have sexual intercourse makes a valid marriage impossible (although the application of this rule to the marriage of an aged person is beset with evident difficulties). However, while the simple ability to perform the act is required, mainstream rotal jurisprudence has consistently refused to endorse any suggestion that the ability to give or derive sexual satisfaction through the act is an essential obligation under c. 1095. Thus, as regards frigidity in a woman (which is not accepted as a form of impotence), even tentative suggestions that it might be regarded as an incapacity for some essential matrimonial obligation under c. 1095(3) have gathered no support.

A homosexual tendency may render the conjugal act less satisfactory to one or both spouses, just as frigidity in the wife does. But (always allowing for the possible relevance of c. 1098) a "less than ideal" ability to perform the act offers no basis for a declaration of consensual incapacity under c. 1095.

Two older persons for whom the physical side of marriage – the actual conjugal act – is of little or practically no interest have the right to marry, even if this lack of interest derives from a rooted homosexual condition that was always present in one or other party.

5. If Church jurisprudence were to hold that any degree of homosexual inclination incapacitates for exercising the legitimate right to marry, this could be held discriminatory also in regard to the rights of homosexuals themselves. It would deprive them of the possibility of marrying someone whom they wish to marry and who, despite their condition, wishes to be united in marriage with them. From the supernatural point of view, they would be deprived of the special sacramental graces of marriage, which are such a powerful help to salvation and holiness.

A psychologist with broad experience in this field writes: "I have had contact with more than one homosexual whose marriage had been a great help in avoiding homosexual adventures and in [avoiding] abandoning himself to other neurotic inclinations. The situation of many married homosexuals is identical with that of other married neurotics. It is sensible to warn a homosexual as well as his future marriage partner of the difficulties they will almost certainly face if they decide to marry, but it must not be an iron rule to discourage such intended marriages."[23]

Conclusion

Christian personalism, given such a prominent place in *Gaudium et Spes* by the Fathers of Vatican II, and so powerfully developed by Pope John Paul II, is rooted in the truth that "man cannot fully find himself except through a sincere gift of himself" (GS, 24). To avoid alienation and indeed total frustration, we need to come out of ourselves, to "lose our life" – in search of higher values and in real service toward others – in order to find it. The confusion about homosexuality is one more outgrowth of the ego-syntonic mentality (the "learning to like oneself" approach) that has been the tonic of psychological thought and therapeutic practice for the past half-century and more.

How far this approach is from the truth about human freedom and fulfillment is a matter that each Christian, and particularly each Christian psychologist or psychiatrist, should be able to judge for himself. In their reflections they could find no better guide than the closing words of Pope John Paul II's Encyclical *Veritatis Splendor*:

> I ask everyone to look more deeply at man, whom Christ has saved in the mystery of his love, and at the human being's unceasing search for truth and meaning. Different philosophical systems have lured people into believing that they are their own absolute master, able to decide their own destiny and future in complete autonomy, trusting only in themselves and their own powers. But this can never be the grandeur of the human being, who can find fulfilment only in choosing to enter the truth, to make a home under the shade of Wisdom and dwell there. Only within this horizon of truth will people understand their freedom in its fullness and their call to know and love God as the supreme realization of their true self.[24]

Endnotes

* Editors note: This chapter is an adapted form of the section on legal considerations, of a sentence of July 9, 1998 of the Roman Rota. The rotal "Turnus," or panel of judges, in that case was presided over by Msgr. Burke, who also wrote the decision.

1 c. Huot, Jan. 28, 1974: R.R. Dec., vol. 66, p. 28. (R.R. Dec. refers to the officially published volumes of rotal decisions. "c" (or "corant") indicates the Presiding judge in the particular case cited.

2 c. Pompedda, Oct. 6, 1969: vol. 61, p. 917.

3 c. Anné, Feb. 6, 1973: vol. 65, p. 64.

4 c. Pompedda, Oct. 19, 1992: vol. 84, p. 496.

5 Pompedda, supra note 2, at 916.

6 c. Serrano, July 18, 1981: vol. 73, p. 423.

7 137 *American Journal of Psychiatry* 890 (1980).

8 "Putting DSM-IV in Perspective," 155 *American Journal of Psychiatry* 159 (1990).

9 J. Eaton, "The Assessment of Mental Health," 108 *American Journal of Psychiatry* 81-90 (1951).

10 Id. at 82.

11 Id. at 89.

12 R Littlewood: "Against Pathology: The New Psychiatry and Its Critics," 159 *British Journal of Psychiatry* 696, 699 (1991)

13 See AAS 79 (1987), 1454-55.

14 *Catechism of the Catholic Church*, nos. 2348, 2337, 2339, 2342.

15 CCC, no. 2357-59.

16 *Veritatis splendor* no. 32.

17 AAS 79 (1987), 1457.

18 DSM-IV, p. xxiii.

19 Id.

20 AAS 79 (1987), 1457.

21 P, Zavalloni, *Elementi di psicopatologia educativa*, 1982, pp. 49–50. A declaration of incapacity for a valid marriage is certainly not justified in the case of an "occasional homosexual."

22 Dr. Eli Coleman: "The Married Lesbian": 14 *Marriage and Family Review* 121, 132 [1989],

23 Gerard J. M. van den Aardweg: *On the Origins and Treatment of Homosexuality*, 147 (Praeger, New York, 1986)

24 VS no. 107.

Morality

Scripture and Homosexuality
Kevin E. Miller

"I live, no longer I, but Christ lives in me; insofar as I now live in the flesh, I live by faith in the Son of God who has loved me and given himself up for me. . . . For you were called for freedom, brothers. But do not use this freedom as an opportunity for the flesh; rather, serve one another through love. . . . I say, then: live by the Spirit and you will certainly not gratify the desire of the flesh. . . . Now those who belong to Christ have crucified their flesh with its pas - sions and desires." – Gal. 2:20; 5:13, 16, 24 (RNAB)

Introduction: Scripture in Church Statements on Homosexual Acts

The Second Vatican Council, in its Decree on Priestly Formation, taught that "students should receive a most careful training in Holy Scripture, which should be the soul, as it were, of all theology," and went on to specify that moral theology "should draw more fully on the teaching of holy Scripture and should throw light upon the exalted vocation of the faithful in Christ and their obligation to bring forth fruit in charity for the life of the world."[1]

Subsequently, a Congregation for the Doctrine of the Faith (CDF) letter has insisted that, contrary to the claims made by "a new exegesis of Sacred Scripture," the Church's teaching that homosexual acts are immoral is truly based on Scripture, and "not on isolated phrases for facile theological argument, but on the solid foundation of a constant Biblical testimony."[2] The CDF explains that the "basic plan" is found in *Genesis* 1–3: "Human beings . . . are nothing less than the work of God himself; and in the complementarity of the sexes, they are called to reflect the inner unity of the creator." However, "this truth about persons being an image of God has been obscured by original sin. There inevitably follows a loss of awareness of the covenantal character of the union these persons had with God and with each other." The CDF next cites *Gen.* 19:1–11, where the "deterioration . . . continues in the story of the men of Sodom. There can be no doubt of the moral judgment made there against homosexual relations." The author of *Lev.* 18:22 and 20:13 "excludes from the People of God those who behave in a homosexual fashion." Similarly, Paul "lists those who behave in a homosexual fashion among those who shall not enter the Kingdom of God" (1 *Cor.* 6:9). Paul also "uses homosexual behaviour as an example of the blindness which has overcome humankind. Instead of the original harmony between Creator and creatures, the acute distortion of idolatry has led to all kinds of moral excess. Paul is at a loss to find a clearer example of this disharmony than homosexual relations" (*Rom.* 1:18–32). Finally, he "explicitly names as sinners those who engage in homosexual acts" (1 *Tim.* 1:10).[3]

The more recent *Catechism of the Catholic Church* has been said to exemplify what the Council had in mind in its call for Scripture to be the soul of theology.[4] The *Catechism* follows the CDF in saying that the Church's teaching concerning homosexual acts is based "on Sacred Scripture, which presents homosexual acts as acts of grave depravity," and citing in support *Gen.* 19:1–29, *Rom.* 1:24–27, 1 *Cor.* 6:10, and 1 *Tim.* 1:10.[5]

The CDF and the *Catechism* do not, however, defend at length their interpretation of the texts they cite concerning homosexual acts. And it is precisely their interpretation that is being called into question by the "new exegesis" to which the CDF refers.[6] In this chapter, I shall provide a defense of the use of Scripture in the CDF letter and the *Catechism*. I shall first discuss in some detail the specific texts cited by the CDF. I shall argue that, contrary to the recent claims that I shall explain at greater length, these texts do condemn homosexual acts in themselves as immoral. Second, I shall address the question of the relevance of these biblical condemnations for Christians today. Specifically, I shall respond to the objection that they are inconsistent with the core of the New Testament message and could therefore be modified today (for example, that homosexual acts by people of "homosexual orientation" could be approved). To accomplish this, I shall look at "the core of the New Testament message" as understood by Paul, and consider how it can help us understand what his moral teaching means. I shall thus show how, in drawing from Scripture in its analysis of homosexual acts, moral theology also responds to the Council's call to "throw light upon the exalted vocation of the faithful in Christ and their obligation to bring forth fruit in charity." For Paul's moral teachings have as their context a most precise understanding of what our "vocation in Christ" is and what it means to "bring forth fruit in charity." At the same time, they do not render irrelevant, and in a sense they presuppose, (philosophical) analysis of the nature of (homo)sexual acts. Finally, I shall explain the CDF's warning – drawing from the Council – that "the interpretation of Scripture must be in substantial accord with [the Church's] Tradition."[7] I shall clarify why we may trust that nothing in Scripture will be at odds with that Tradition, and why we may use Tradition to shed further light on Scripture and confirm what we take to follow about homosexual acts from Paul's principles about Christian life.

I
The Scriptural Texts

All five texts cited by the CDF – the Sodom story, the condemnations in *Leviticus*, and the teachings of Paul in *Romans*, 1 *Corinthians*, and 1 *Timothy* – have been subjected to revisionist interpretation in recent years. Scholars have argued that they are not intended to represent more than cultural norms or that the acts they condemn do not include at least some homosexual acts. I shall here present these contentions in more detail and offer some initial responses, arguing that they are not well-founded.

A. The Sodom story

It has recently been claimed that the story of Sodom in *Genesis* 19 not only has nothing to do with homosexual acts, but more generally has nothing to do with sexual morality at all. This claim has been argued in two ways. The more radical claim, elaborated perhaps first by Derrick Sherwin Bailey, is that when the people of Sodom tell Lot to bring his (unbeknownst to them, angelic) visitors out so that the people may "know" them (*Gen.* 19:5 – the RNAB translates the Hebrew as "have intimacies with"), the word "know" has only its literal meaning (as is usually the case in the Old Testament) rather than its "biblical" meaning of sexual contact (as in only ten clear cases in the OT, as well as the famous case of Mary's words in *Luke* 1:34, "How can this be, since I do not know [RNAB: I have no relations with a] man?"). Instead of demanding (homo)sexual contact with the visitors, so this claim goes, the people of Sodom are only asking to make the visitors' acquaintance. But why would they be so insistent about this as to try to break down Lot's door (*Gen.* 19:9)? It has been hypothesized that since Lot was himself not a citizen of Sodom (13:12), he had no right to bring guests into the city without introducing them to the citizens.

However, there are problems with this line of interpretation. First, it must somehow be explained why, then, what the people of Sodom did was so evil. Bailey says that it would have been contrary to Lot's obligation of hospitality.[8] The problem with this is that Lot could presumably have introduced his visitors to the people without violating his obligations as a host, and therefore, if his refusal to do so exceeded his rights in Sodom, he would hardly have been justified in calling the people's request a "wicked thing" (19:7). Bailey's interpretation, then, seems self-contradictory.

It must also be explained why Lot would have offered his daughters to the people as a substitute for the male visitors. Bailey claims that "its connexion with the purpose (whatever it was) for which the citizens demanded the production of his guests is purely imaginary. No doubt the surrender of his daughters was simply the most tempting bribe that Lot could offer on the spur of the moment to appease the hostile crowd."[9] However, Lot's offer seems clearly to "recogni[ze] that the crowd is motivated not by curiosity about the guests' origins but by desire for erotic experience." Furthermore, Lot describes his daughters as not having "known" (RNAB: "had intercourse with") man (19:8). Here, the "biblical" sense of the word is obviously intended, supporting the standard reading of the same word as having the same sense in the citizens' demand just three verses earlier.[10]

A less radical claim about the Sodom story is that, while the people are indeed demanding sexual contact with Lot's guests, it is not the homosexual nature of that contact that would be wicked, but rather any sexual contact with guests, insofar as that would be, again, a violation of hospitality, perhaps all the more grave since the guests were messengers from God.[11] Perhaps the basic problem with this claim is that it is wholly speculative – if the text does not explicitly say that it is the homosexual nature of the proposed conduct that is wicked, neither does it deny this.

The fact that other Scriptural references to the Sodom story do not refer to the proposed homosexual conduct itself as the wickedness is adduced as evidence for the revisionist interpretation, but this is not telling. First, to the extent that other texts speak of Sodom's lack of social justice, it must be remembered that "[p]rophetic writings rarely recapitulate events or actions described in older sacred texts. Instead they remind audiences that the obvious sins and punishments . . . result from the less readily recognized sins that a later generation shares. Thus *Ezechiel* 16:46–51 attributes Sodom's sexual licentiousness to its general climate of luxury and self-indulgence."[12]

Second, if the people's request is a failure of hospitality and/or an act of rejection of guests or of God's messengers, it must be explained in precisely what way their proposed conduct is inhospitable or a rejection. This point is sharpened when one recalls that Lot thought it would be preferable for the people to "know" his daughters. It is difficult to understand why coerced heterosexual contact with a resident alien's daughters is less inhospitable, or less of a rejection of him and his family, than coerced homosexual contact with his guests would be – unless one assumes that homosexual contact is more radically a violation of one's dignity as a person than heterosexual contact. The only alternative would seem to be an appeal to "the low status of female children in the society," but to say that is all there is to it is again wholly speculative, and a reading on which "[t]he story [would have] no continuity at this point"; thus the argument can be called "special pleading."[13]

B. Leviticus: The "Holiness Code" and "Abominations"

The other Old Testament passages cited by the CDF as explicit condemnations of homosexual acts are the prohibitions of such acts in *Lev.* 18:22, "You shall not lie with a male as with a woman; such a thing is an abomination," and 20:13, which specifies the death penalty for this act. It is, in fact, undisputed that there is here a reference to homosexual acts. However, the meaning of the condemnation of such an act as an "abomination" is disputed. *Leviticus* 18 begins, "The Lord said to Moses, 'Speak to the Israelites and tell them: I, the Lord, am your God. You shall not do as they do in the land of Egypt, where you once lived, nor shall you do as they do in the land of Canaan, where I am bringing you; do not conform to their customs. My decrees you shall carry out . . .'" (vv. 1–4). The "Holiness Code" that follows, it is argued, prohibits not actions that are intrinsically or by nature evil, but rather actions that are contrary to the customs and identity of the People of God at this time. The word "abomination" is said to signify this.[14]

However, this interpretation is not borne out by a careful look at the Holiness Code and by the actions called "abominations" in the Old Testament. The provisions of the Code in Leviticus 18 prohibit not only homosexual acts but also such acts as incest, adultery, immolating children to Molech, and bestiality. Presumably these are not opposed merely to Israelite custom. Furthermore, Lev. 18:26 prohibits not only Israelites but also "resident aliens" from performing these acts, which is not consistent with the hypothesis that it is Israelite identity that is at issue. The word "abomination" is used in the Old Testament for idolatry as well as such acts as "infanticide, consulting fortune tellers and invoking ghosts." It is not, however, used for violations of dietary laws (although in one place it is used for the animals which may not be eaten, as opposed to the action of eating them).[15] If, then, some actions that seem to be more than betrayals of one's identity as an Israelite are called "abominations," and actions that do not seem to be more than this are not, what does the word mean – what do "abominations" have in common; what is their essence?

Lynn Boughton, author of a superb article on the biblical treatment of homosexuality, writes:

> It seems . . . that the act must involve treating a person or object in a way that contradicts its fundamental nature. For example . . . worship of idols is [an abomination] because such acts of worship deny that there is only one God and deny the inanimate nature of idols. . . . [T]he worship of false gods by sacrificing one's children is [an abomination] because one ends a true, self-identifying relationship and a real life for an imaginary relationship for something that has no life. . . .

> Similarly . . . ["abomination"] describes a group of actions including infanticide, consulting fortune tellers and invoking ghosts. This grouping of "abominations" indicates that more is at stake than violation of cultural identity or ritual purity. What these acts have in common is either attributing to a person a power or identity he does not have . . . or denying the human identity of one's offspring. . . .

> The specifically sexual prohibitions of the Torah seem to be consistent with this principle of respecting the physical identity of what God has created. Since the physical manifestations of gender are created by God and seem to have some special significance in human relationships . . . it is an abomination to dissociate genital acts from the physical or relational identity of a man or a woman. . . .

> In this large . . . context the laws in *Lev.* 18:22 and 20:13 . . . are not mere prohibitions of ritual uncleanness. Instead, denial of a person's sexual physiology is a violation of a much more fundamental or moral

law, because, though it may be in accord with a person's desires, it rejects a person's God-given gender.[16]

Bailey, who denies that the Sodom story is about (homo)sexuality, concurs in this analysis of the *Leviticus* texts:

> ["Abomination"], as we have seen, is closely associated with idolatry, and designates not only false gods but also the worship and conduct of those who serve them. By a natural extension of meaning, however, it can also denote whatever reverses the proper order of things, and this seems to be the connotation of ["abomination"] as applied to homosexual acts in *Leviticus*. Such acts are regarded as "abomination" . . . because, as a reversal of what is sexually natural, they exemplify the spirit of idolatry which is itself the fundamental subversion of true order.[17]

Hence, those performing homosexual acts are excluded from the People of God because of the immoral nature of the acts, not because they are not customary or accepted. This analysis of the *Leviticus* passages, it should be noted, also serves to defend the CDF's treatment of the story of the creation of male and female as relevant to the issue of homosexual acts, which has also been questioned.[18]

C. 1 Corinthians and 1 Timothy: Pauline condemnations

We may turn now to the New Testament, beginning with *1 Cor.* 6:9 and *1 Tim.* 1:10, which use similar language. First *Corinthians* refers to *malakoi* and *arsenokoitai,* saying that neither will inherit the kingdom of God. First *Timothy* counts *arsenokoitai* among those who are "lawless and unruly, godless and sinful, unholy and profane" (1:9). The dispute about these passages concerns the meaning of *malakoi* and *arsenokoitai*. The first of these Greek words denotes softness or even effeminacy. It has been suggested that it does not refer specifically to homosexual acts but to sexual or moral looseness or laxity in general.[19] Those who question whether Scripture prohibits homosexuality have treated *arsenokoitai* in various ways. One argument is that it refers to male prostitutes – including heterosexual male prostitutes.[20] Another, however, grants that it is "some kind of reference to male same-sex acts," but in effect denies that Paul intended these texts as moral condemnations, just as the condemnations in *Leviticus* are said not to have been moral condemnations, as discussed above.[21]

What do these words mean? In classical Greek in general, "in reference to people, the term [*malakoi*] designates the adoption of a passive, feminine role in physical relations"; for example, Aristotle and Plato use the word to refer to men who act in a feminine manner or specifically to the receptive partners in male homosexual acts.[22] It is gratuitous to deny that Paul could have intended this meaning. And given the pairing of this word with *arsenokoitai*, which I shall discuss next, it seems the more likely meaning.

Arsenokoitai does seem to refer to the active partners in male homosexual acts. It comes from the Greek words meaning "man" ("male") and "to lie." The latter verb, in the Bible, refers to "the active male role of impregnating or seeding," and the corresponding noun is used by Paul to mean "intercourse." In general, when this word is part of a compound, "the first part of the compound is the object, not the subject"[23] – thus, *arsenokoitai* would be "those who lie as a man *with a man*," not "men who lie as a man (with either a man or a woman)."[24] And again, the pairing of this word with *malakoi*, which plausibly, indeed most plausibly, means passive male homosexual partners, strengthens the case still more.

The argument that Paul's references to *arsenokoitai* are not intended as moral condemnations takes them to be part of standard lists of sins, related to those discussed above in *Leviticus*, reflecting cultural concerns. Did Paul,[25] wittingly or unwittingly, include in his letters such apparently severe condemnations of acts that are not intrinsically evil? It is unlikely that Paul did not intend by his words to describe these acts as intrinsically evil, for the reasons adduced in the discussion of *Leviticus*. That is, granting that Paul is saying something similar to what was being said in *Leviticus*, if the revisionists are wrong about *Leviticus*, then they are wrong about Paul, too. To say that an act excludes one from the Kingdom of God is to say something about the nature of the act, not about arbitrary prejudices. And it is unlikely that Paul – as aware as he was of the priority for Christians of grace over law, to be discussed in the second part of this chapter – would not have considered carefully whether a particular prohibition does or does not reflect the nature of an action. Indeed, when he prohibits something only on the basis of his own judgment, or primarily as contrary to custom or good order, he is generally careful to clarify this (cf. *1 Cor.* 7:25, 11:16).

D. Romans: *"Unnatural" desires and acts*

The final New Testament text that must be considered is *Rom.* 1:24–27. There, Paul says of those who worshiped creatures rather than the Creator that "[t]heir females exchanged natural relations for unnatural, and the males likewise gave up natural relations with females and burned with lust for one another. Males did shameful things with males and thus received in their own persons the due penalty for their perversity." The primary issue about this text arises out of Paul's description of homosexual desires and acts as "unnatural." To exactly which homosexual desires/acts is he referring, and what moral assessment does he intend?

It has been suggested, first, that Paul is speaking only of homosexuality that is contrary to someone's "personal nature," that is, homosexual desires or acts, presumably in an orgiastic spirit, perhaps as part of an idolatrous ritual, on the part of someone who we would call today a heterosexual.[26] This is, however, another example of speculation that, if not inconsistent with the text, is nonetheless not grounded in it. It cannot be proved that Paul only considers homosexual acts "unnatural" when performed by heterosexuals.

Furthermore, this interpretation would actually empty Paul's words of meaning. It is difficult to imagine someone choosing to perform any sexual act for which he or she did not have some desire, even if a desire to some degree elicited by the circumstances. If someone desires in any way homosexual acts, what bearing does the fact that the person also has or has had heterosexual desires have on the question of whether the homosexual desires are contrary to the person's "personal nature"?

Finally, this interpretation is sometimes supported with the claim that Paul would not have been aware of the existence of "homosexuals" in the modern sense – people with primarily or exclusively homosexual desires, for whom these desires and the corresponding acts might therefore, in some sense, not be contrary to nature.[27] But as Bailey recognizes, "St. Paul's words can only be understood in the sense which he himself would have attached to them, without introducing distinctions which he did not intend, and which would have been unintelligible to him."[28] That is, the argument that St. Paul was unaware that some people's "personal nature" is homosexual begs the question of what his response would have been had he known of, or spoken explicitly of, such people. It needs to be further argued, not merely assumed, that he would have approved of their homosexual acts. And for reasons I shall discuss both in the next paragraph and in the second part of this chapter, this is unlikely.

Second, the question has been raised of exactly what Paul is trying to say about those of whom he is speaking in this passage. It has been claimed that "the point of the passage is not to stigmatize sexual behavior of any sort but to condemn the Gentiles for their general infidelity."[29] It is arguable that "general infidelity" is the primary concern of the passage (and the CDF's characterization of the passage recognizes this). However, it is important to consider the precise relationship posited by Paul between this general infidelity and homosexual acts. The acts are in some sense a consequence of infidelity, of having "exchanged the truth of God for a lie and revered and worshiped the creature rather than the Creator" (v. 25). For Paul continues: "*Therefore*, God handed them over to degrading passions . . ." (v. 26). Setting aside the question of the sense of God's agency, the "passions" are clearly presented as undesirable and as a kind of punishment or consequence of evil. Thus, even though they are not the evil with which the passage is primarily concerned, they are, surely, "stigmatized." (One can also note the other kinds of punishments mentioned in vv.

28–31, parallel to vv. 24–27, and consider that "wickedness, evil, greed, and malice" are presumably "stigmatized," even if they are no more the primary concern here than are homosexual passions/acts.)

Does Paul give any indication of what is intrinsically wrong with the passions, or does he only say they are wrong and describe them as a punishment? Again, Paul calls them "unnatural." It is claimed that this word lacks moral significance for Paul. What gives color to this argument is Paul's description later in *Romans* of the Gentiles' salvation (their being "grafted" into the "cultivated tree" of God's People) as something "contrary to nature" (11:24; the Greek phrase is the same as that translated above by "unnatural"). Clearly, Paul does not mean in that passage that it is immoral for God to save the Gentiles.[30] However, it seems that the word "nature" has a different sense in the latter passage, which expressly distinguishes between what is natural for Jews and what is natural for Gentiles, at the service of an argument that if the Gentiles can be saved, so, *a fortiori,* can the Jews, and if the Jews can be cut off from salvation, so, *a fortiori,* can the Gentiles. In this latter passage, it seems, Paul is indeed using the word "nature" in a sense different from the philosophical sense familiar from natural law theory. But this does not mean that Paul never used the word in anything like this philosophical sense. Something like that sense does seem to be intended in *Romans* 1.[31]

In fact, though, the meanings of "nature" in *Romans* 1 and *Romans* 11 have something in common. In each case, the word has something to do with God's plan. In *Romans* 1, when people turn away from God, they cease to act in accordance with his plan. In *Romans* 11, God's plan as it had played out in the Old Testament included the cultivation of the Jews alone into God's people; now, "contrary to" that plan, God "grafts" the Gentiles, too, into that "cultivated tree." In the latter case, the plan as it was known to the Jews was not yet complete. In the former case, there is no indication that Paul thought that God had changed his plan for human sexuality, and every indication that he had not, given that he "stigmatizes" the "unnatural" desires and behavior of which he speaks. Indeed, we have in *Romans* 1 a treatment of the relationship between homosexual desires and God's plan much like that in *Leviticus*, as discussed above.

II. The Christian Context

Granting that, as I have argued, all these texts are best read as intending to condemn homosexual acts, and to condemn them as intrinsically evil because they are contrary to God's plan as manifest in creation, the question remains of their relevance for the Christian vocation. Put differently, it needs still to be shown whether and how homosexual acts are contrary to the New Testament message about salvation. For, it has, in effect, been argued, undue concern with the created order is itself contrary to the Christian message. According to that message, what is important is not what kind of action one performs (that is, how it is related to the created order) but the attitude with which one performs it.[32] (Indeed, a presupposition of this sort is perhaps at the root of the difficulty some commentators have in thinking Paul could ascribe moral significance to "nature.") With regard to sexuality specifically, the argument is that Paul "would have disapproved of any form of sexuality which had as its end purely sexual pleasure, and he might have disapproved of relationships directed chiefly at the expression of erotic passion"; "Christian sexuality was . . . a question of good stewardship – of using sexuality in a way that was not obsessive . . . did not cause scandal, and did not distract Christians from the service of the Lord"; thus, Paul "clearly regarded licit sexuality as that contained within a permanent and monogamous relationship" – these being the criteria for "loving" sexuality – and, finally, "[t]here is no inherent reason why unions between persons of the same sex could not have met these moral criteria."[33] (This would, presumably, be possible especially between persons of "homosexual orientation.") And if, as I have argued, Paul did condemn homosexual acts as intrinsically evil, this is only because Paul was in those places untrue to his own Christian moral principles.

Whatever one takes this argument to undermine – my interpretation of the texts in themselves, or their significance within the Bible taken as a whole and read in a Christian manner – it does raise the profound question of the relationship between the orders of creation and redemption, and deserves some response for that reason as well as because of its practical importance. I shall offer that response by looking briefly at Paul's most extensive treatment of Christian freedom, the *Letter to the Galatians*. In this letter, Paul addresses a community of Gentile Christians whom he had evangelized, and who have since been persuaded by some group to follow such Jewish laws as circumcision. Paul makes no secret of his anger – he omits the prayer of thanksgiving for something about his addressees that is usually included near the beginning of his letters; he calls the Galatians "stupid" (3:1); and he calls those to whom the Galatians have been listening "accursed" (1:9) and wishes that they "might also castrate themselves" (5:12). Paul argues extensively and intensively that the example he gave the Galatians was one of faith, not observance of the law; that their own reception of the Spirit was the result of faith, not works of the law; that the Old Testament, rightly understood in the light of Christ, witnesses to the primacy of faith rather than law; and that to observe the law is to fall from sonship in Christ and the Spirit back into slavery.

At the same time, Paul exhorts the Galatians: "[D]o not use this freedom as an opportunity for the flesh; rather, serve one another through love.'" (5:13). He then proceeds to speak of certain rather specific actions as incompatible with love, and other actions as compatible with love. Is he thus reintroducing the arbitrary restrictions he has just argued to be of no benefit and, indeed, destructive? By no means. In Paul's initial discussion of his own faith and that of the Galatians, he has already made clear that there is a connection between the life of faith and the action of Christ and the Spirit. Of his own conversion and initial faith, he says that God "was pleased to reveal His Son *in* me" (1:16 – not "to me," as in the RNAB and some other translations). It was this revelation of Christ *in* Paul, through his faith, that formed the basis for his preaching. Paul sums up his own life of faith: "I live, no longer I, but Christ lives in me; insofar as I now live in the flesh, I live by faith in the Son of God who has loved me and given Himself up for me" (2:20). Paul here refers, not only to Christ, not only to Christ's love as though a disincarnate "attitude," but also to the specific action of having "given himself up" in which Christ's love was incarnate.[34] Paul's own life of faith is, in short, by its very nature inseparable from his allowing Christ to live through him by Paul's acting – in specific ways – in union with Christ's love. Paul then goes on to speak of the faith in which the Galatians had initially imitated his own, and of their reception of the Spirit from their faith (3:2). Faith, then, is openness to the loving actions of both Christ and the Spirit. This forms the basis for Paul's exhortations to "live by the Spirit" (5:16) and "crucif[y] their flesh" with Christ (5:24) through specific acts of love.

Now, this presupposes that, while the actions for which Paul is reprimanding the Galatians – circumcision, perhaps adherence to dietary laws or celebration of certain feasts – are of no intrinsic value, are not intrinsically necessary for a life of faith through love, some kinds of actions (or omissions) – those discussed in 5:19–22 – are. If this is true, it is evident that the claims about the irrelevancy of particular kinds of actions that serve as the basis for the dismissal of the possibility that Paul condemns homosexual acts are gratuitous. At the very least, Paul was not being untrue to his own principles in condemning such acts, and the condemnations are not made doubtful or irrelevant by putting them in the context of Paul's (or the New Testament's) message as a whole.

But the question then becomes: How do we know what kinds of actions are, like Christ's Sacrifice, acts of love, and what kinds are incompatible with love? Are these categorizations intelligible? It is at this point that we can return to the order of nature or creation. Christian love can certainly exceed respect for the way in which God created us. What it cannot intelligibly do is deny this. A love that did not respect this would not be a love for *us*. Thus, most generally, God's love for us, in making us his sons and daughters (*Gal.* 4:4), indeed in making us sharers in his own nature (2 *Pt.* 1:4), raises us above what we were made in creation. But while making us more than human, it does not negate what is good about our humanity.[35] Thus also, we as Christians are called to treat one another not merely as human beings, but as beings called to a supernatural destiny – more generously, that is, than the good of our human nature in itself demands; with loving mercy, not only with mere justice.[36] But this cannot involve treating each other with less respect than that demanded by our nature, by justice.

The demands of love that go beyond justice can only be known by revelation; Christ's commandment, "Love one another as I love you" (*John* 15:12), exceeds what is known about morality from the Old Testament, let alone from philosophical reflection. But the minimal demands of justice, what is necessary minimally to respect each other as (created) human persons, can be known using human reason. It is indeed human reason, of the sort known as natural-law reasoning, that is necessary to begin to make intelligible Paul's condemnation of homosexual acts, even in a Christian context, even though only that context makes fully clear the consequences of such acts (they are contrary not only to the good of our humanity, but also, therefore, to that humanity's participation in the good of God's own life).[37]

It is worth noting here a point illustrated by what I have said: making Scripture the "soul" of theology and using it to throw light upon our vocation to charity in Christ does not mean making Biblical theology the whole of theology, nor even dismissing moral philosophy as irrelevant to moral theology, as some critics of the Church's use of the Scriptural texts I have discussed seem to presuppose. In the end, natural-law reasoning, for example about sexual acts, is invaluable in understanding what Scripture says about morality, for example about those same acts.

Why are homosexual acts contrary to "nature" or "natural law"? Full treatment of this question is beyond the scope of this chapter. The observation that God did make humans "male and female" is only the beginning of an answer; it needs further to be specified in what morally relevant sense only males and females are complementary (rather than males and males or females and females), and the CDF's appeal to *Genesis* 1–3 presupposes such an explanation. By way of summary, however, it can be pointed out that, at least with regard to procreation, males complement only females, and vice-versa; that our procreative potential is no mere physical or biological "fact" but a good, something of value; that to treat our sexuality or genitality as primarily a source of pleasure is to treat this good as though it were not a good or less a good than it is; and, further, that this cannot serve as the foundation for a truly unifying relationship, a relationship of love in even a purely human sense, but only for one of mutual use, itself therefore contrary to our nature as beings with intellect and will.[38] And it should be noted that this argument would apply regardless of the "sexual orientation" of the person performing the acts. The argument shows that the acts are by their nature not compatible with love; the disposition of the person performing them does not change their nature in a way that would affect the argument.

III. Scripture and Tradition

I would like, finally, to explain and defend the CDF's statement that Scripture must be interpreted in accord with the Church's Tradition. For it is by so interpreting Scripture that even someone who may not grasp fully the intelligibility of, say, Scriptural condemnations of homosexual acts, can nonetheless be confident that such acts are incompatible with Christian life. Thus, even if my historical-critical arguments about the meaning of the texts discussed are not fully conclusive, one can properly say that those texts do condemn homosexual acts; indeed, one can go further and say that arguments that purport to show that Scripture supports the morality of homosexual acts cannot possibly be sound. Why is this?

First of all, Scripture is inspired by God. This does not mean that God dictates every word of Scripture (surely in some cases – see, e.g., *Luke* 1:1–4 – the authors were unaware of inspiration in any sense, let alone dictation; and some texts – e.g., *1 Cor.* 1:14–16 – seem to evince the limitations of a human mind and therefore to be incompatible with crude understandings of inspiration). Nor does it excuse Christians from being careful to read texts in the context of the whole canon of Scripture, not in isolation. In fact, Scripture witnesses to the People of God's gradual understanding of God and his plan as he gradually revealed these to them, culminating only in the sending of the Incarnate Word.[39] Nonetheless, inspiration does at least mean that what is recorded in Scripture is what God wanted recorded; indeed, God can be called the author of Scripture.[40]

Second, Scripture does not exhaust what God has done to provide for the transmission to future ages of the interventions in human history by which God revealed Himself. The transmission of the Gospel in the Church through the preaching of the Apostles and their successors, the bishops, is also protected by the Holy Spirit.[41]

What follows from this? When a human author has written multiple works about the same subject, it is often necessary to interpret them in light of each other, to allow each to shed light on a different facet of their subject matter and therefore also on each other. In the same way, God is the author of all of Scripture as well as what is passed on in Tradition. It is therefore necessary not only to treat Scripture as a unity, but to treat Scripture and Tradition together as a unity. Where the meaning or significance of something in Scripture is unclear, Tradition can often shed light on the subject.[42] And the Christian faith includes confidence that it is impossible that Scripture and Tradition could contradict each other. To deny this is to deny the action of the Holy Spirit in Scripture and Tradition – the very sources of what we hold by faith, the very basis for our faith.

Hence, it is unfair to the CDF to assert that, in view of revisionist arguments, "the passages [mentioned by the CDF] are complex enough to warrant more than a couple of paragraphs. If the recent scholarship is going to be called 'gravely erroneous,' then it ought to be addressed. Further, it should be refuted if possible by better scholarship. Dismissing it out of hand and interpreting Scripture by way of conclusionary statements is intellectually dishonest and pastorally unjust."[43] Scripture scholarship is necessary to the Church. Scripture sheds light on Tradition as much as vice-versa, and Scripture scholars have done much, and can do much more, to elucidate texts and thereby prepare for the reading of Scripture and Tradition in each other's light. As but one example, they have an invaluable contribution to make in seeking an ever-deeper understanding of the passages I have discussed, one which will show even more clearly the harmony between them and Tradition. But it is unreasonable to expect a document of the nature of the CDF's to engage in detail the different and changing claims of scholars, and it is theologically incorrect to claim that any other procedure is "intellectually dishonest."

Conclusions

I have in this chapter taken up the use of Scripture in the CDF's "Letter to the Bishops of the Catholic Church on the Pastoral Care of Homosexual Persons" as an opening into the subject of what Scripture says about homosexuality. I have argued, contrary to contemporary revisionist interpretations, that the Old and New Testament passages the CDF cites do indeed condemn homosexual acts; that they are consistent with and indeed presupposed by the core of the New Testament message about our vocation to charity in Christ, because homosexual acts are by their nature incompatible with that vocation; and that it is intellectually and pastorally sensible to refer to the Tradition of the Church to support this reading. Catholics can be sure that the CDF's approach and conclusions are grounded in solid Catholic Scripture scholarship, as envisioned by Vatican II, and that arguments that Scripture does not condemn homosexual acts (or even supports them) are unfounded.

Endnotes

1. Second Vatican Council, Decree on Priestly Formation *Optatam Totius* (1965), trans. B. Hayes, et al., no. 16, in A. Flannery, ed., *Vatican Collection, vol. 1: Vatican Council II: The Conciliar and Postconciliar Documents* (Northport, NY: Costello, 1992).

2. Congregation for the Doctrine of the Faith, "Letter to the Bishops of the Catholic Church on the Pastoral Care of Homosexual Persons" (Washington, DC: USCC, 1986), nos. 4–5.

3. Congregation for the Doctrine of the Faith, "Pastoral Care," no. 6.

4. For a general defense of the *Catechism*'s use of Scripture, see William S. Kurz and Kevin E. Miller, "The Use of Scripture in the *Catechism of the Catholic Church*," *Communio* 23 (1996): 480–507. For its use of

Kevin E. Miller

Scripture in its treatment of morality in particular, see Servais Pinckaers, "The Use of Scripture and the Renewal of Moral Theology: The *Catechism* and *Veritatis Splendor*," *The Thomist* 59 (1995): 1–19.

5. *Catechism of the Catholic Church* (USCC   Libreria Editrice Vaticana, 1994), no. 2357 and n. 140. Cf. also the *Catechism*'s treatments of the Genesis creation and fall narratives (nos. 374–76, 397–401) and its application of the creation narrative to sexual morality (no. 2331) as the context for what it says about homosexuality.

6. In fact, there has been at least one direct response to the CDF's "Letter" citing revisionist scholarship: Dan Grippo, "The Vatican Can Slight Scripture for Its Purpose," in *The Vatican and Homosexuality: Reactions to the "Letter to the Bishops of the Catholic Church on the Pastoral Care of Homosexual Persons,"* ed. Jeannine Gramick and Pat Furey (New York: Crossroad, 1988), 33–39.

7. Congregation for the Doctrine of the Faith, "Pastoral Care," no. 5; Second Vatican Council, Dogmatic Constitution on Divine Revelation *Dei Verbum*, no. 10. Cf. also ibid., no. 12, and the *Catechism*, nos. 95, 113.

8. Derrick Sherwin Bailey, *Homosexuality and the Western Christian Tradition* (Hamden, Conn: Archon, 1975), 2–5.

9. Bailey, *Homosexuality*, 6.

10. Lynn C. Boughton, "Biblical Texts and Homosexuality: A Response to John Boswell," *Irish Theological Quarterly* 58 (1992), 142.

11. Daniel A. Helminiak, *What the Bible* Really *Says about Homosexuality* (San Francisco: Alamo Square Press, 1994), 40.

12. Boughton, "Biblical Texts and Homosexuality," 143.

13. Glenn W. Olsen, "The Gay Middle Ages: A Response to Professor Boswell," *Communio* 8 (1981), 131–32.

14. John Boswell, *Christianity, Social Tolerance, and Homosexuality: Gay People in Western Europe from the Beginning of the Christian Era to the Fourteenth Century* (Chicago and London: Univ. of Chicago Press, 1980), 100–101; Helminiak, *What the Bible* Really *Says*, 45–52.

15. Boughton, "Biblical Texts and Homosexuality," 144–45.

16. Boughton, "Biblical Texts and Homosexuality," 145–46.

17. Bailey, *Homosexuality*, 59–60.

18. Helminiak, *What the Bible* Really *Says*, 100–102.

19. Boswell, *Christianity, Social Tolerance, and Homosexuality,* 106–7; Helminiak, *What the Bible* Really *Says,* 88-89.

20. Boswell, *Christianity, Social Tolerance, and Homosexuality,* 107.

21. Helminiak, *What the Bible* Really *Says,* 85, 91, 92–93.

22. Boughton, "Biblical Texts and Homosexuality," 149.

23. Boughton, "Biblical Texts and Homosexuality," 149–50.

24. The RNAB translates *malakoi* as "boy prostitutes," which captures the notion of passive male homosexual partners but is probably overly narrow.

25. The Pauline authorship of *1 Timothy* is disputed, but at least the condemnation in *1 Corinthians* is certainly Paul's. For a helpful and nuanced discussion of the disputes about the Pauline corpus, see Luke T. Johnson, *The Writings of the New Testament: An Interpretation* (Philadelphia: Fortress, 1986), 255–57, and for *1 Timothy* and the Pastorals specifically, 381–89.

26. Boswell, *Christianity, Social Tolerance, and Homosexuality,* 110–11.

27. On whether there really is a fixed "homosexual orientation," see Jeffrey Satinover, *Homosexuality and the Politics of Truth* (Grand Rapids: Baker, 1996).

28. Bailey, *Homosexuality,* 38.

29. Boswell, *Christianity, Social Tolerance, and Homosexuality,* 108; cf. Helminiak, *What the Bible* Really *Says,* 73–82.

30. Boswell, *Christianity, Social Tolerance, and Homosexuality,* 112.

31. Cf. Olsen, "The Gay Middle Ages," 133–34.

32. Grippo, "The Vatican Can Slight Scripture," 39.

33. Boswell, *Christianity, Social Tolerance, and Homosexuality,* 115–16.

34. For more on the relationship between Christ's actions and his love, see Robert Sokolowski, *Eucharistic Presence: A Study in the Theology of Disclosure* (Washington, DC: Catholic Univ. of America Press, 1994), 62–64.

35. In fact, this is why openness to a share in God's life must itself be a part of our human nature. See Henri de Lubac, *The Mystery of the Supernatural,* trans. Rosemary Sheed (New York: Crossroad, 1998), 53–74.

36. This is, for example, the foundation for John Paul II's teaching on capital punishment; see Kevin E. Miller, "The Role of Mercy in a Culture of Life: John Paul II on Capital Punishment," in *Life and*

Learning VIII, ed. Joseph W. Koterski (Washington, DC: University Faculty for Life, 1999), 405–42.

37. Cf. the CDF, "Declaration on Certain Questions Concerning Sexual Ethics" (Boston: St. Paul Books & Media, 1975), nos. 3–4: "[T]here can be no true promotion of man's dignity unless the essential order of his nature is respected. . . . [I]n fact, divine Revelation and, in its own proper order, philosophical wisdom, emphasize the authentic exigencies of human nature."

38. Cf. Karol Wojtyla's (Pope John Paul II's) natural-law argument against contraception in *Love and Responsibility,* trans. H. T. Willetts (San Francisco: Ignatius Press, 1993), and my summary of this argument, drawing also from some of Wojtlya's essays, in "The Incompatibility of Contraception with Respect for Life," in *Life and Learning VII,* ed. Joseph W. Koterski, S.J. (Washington, DC: University Faculty for Life, 1998), 86–97. Homosexual acts are analogous to contracepted heterosexual acts. Cf. the CDF, "Declaration," no. 8: "[H]omosexual relations are acts which lack an essential and indispensable finality"; and the CDF, "Letter," no. 7: "Homosexual activity is not a complementary union, able to transmit life; and so it thwarts the call to a life of that form of self-giving which the Gospel says is the essence of Christian living. This does not mean that homosexual persons are not often generous and giving of themselves; but when they engage in homosexual activity they confirm within themselves a disordered sexual inclination which is essentially self-indulgent."

39. Cf. Pope John Paul II's treatment of the provisions for capital and corporal punishment in the Old Testament, in *Evangelium Vitae* (1995), no. 40.

40. Second Vatican Council, *Dei Verbum,* no. 11; *Catechism,* nos. 105–106. For further discussion of "inspiration," see Joseph T. Lienhard, *The Bible, the Church, and Authority: The Canon of the Christian Bible in History and Theology* (Collegeville, Minn.: Liturgical Press, 1995), 73–86.

41. Second Vatican Council, *Dei Verbum,* no. 9; *Catechism,* nos. 81–82.

42. For more on the steps involved in the interpretation of Scripture, see Kurz and Miller, "The Use of Scripture," 490–500. For further helpful discussion of the foundations of this, see Sokolowski, *Eucharistic Presence,* 148–50.

43. Grippo, "The Vatican Can Slight Scripture," 39.

The Theology of Hetero- and Homosexuality

Rev. Benedict Ashley, O.P.

The wisdom that comes from above is first of all pure, then peaceable, gentle, compliant, full of mercy and good fruits, without inconstancy or insincerity. (Jm 3: 17).

The Greek term *eupeithes* rendered in this text as "compliant" can also be translated "rich in sympathy." Hence theology, faith seeking understanding, must meditate on the Word of God in a spirit "rich in sympathy," both for the Word's inner meaning and also for those to whom the Word is addressed but who resist it.

Why we are sexual? God said a great deal about that question in the Old Testament, beginning with the two stories of creation in Genesis; so much, in fact, that the New Testament has little to add. Yet Jesus did make one very important pronouncement on marriage and divorce, to which St. Paul refers (I *Cor* 7: 10–11) and which is related at length in *Mark* and *Matthew*. In answer to the Pharisees' question as to what grounds justify a husband in giving his wife the bill of divorcement required by the Law of Moses, Jesus replied,

> Because of the hardness of your hearts he [Moses] wrote this commandment. But from the beginning of creation 'God made them male and female.' For this reason a man shall leave his father and mother and the two shall become one flesh. So they are no longer two but one flesh. Therefore what God has joined together, no human being must separate. Whoever

> divorces his wife and marries another commits adultery against her, and if she divorces her husband and marries another, she commits adultery. (*Mk* 10: 1–1 2; *Mt* 19:3–9)

Matthew then adds,

> His disciples said to him, "If that is the case of a man with his wife, it is better not to marry." He answered, "Not all can accept this word, but only those to whom that is granted. Some are incapable of marriage because they were born so; some, because they were made so by others; some because they have renounced marriage for the sake of the kingdom of heaven. Whoever can accept this ought to accept it."

On another occasion, also, the disciples found His teaching – this time on the Eucharist – much too hard,

> As a result of this, many of His disciples returned to their former way of life and no longer accompanied Him. Jesus then said to the Twelve, "Do you also want to leave?" Simon Peter answered Him, "Master to whom shall we go? You have the words of eternal life. We have come to believe and are convinced that you are the Holy One of God." (Jn 6:66–69)

Note that Jesus by these answers did not condemn, nor did He exclude, anyone from his respect and love. But He was saying that to be His disciple, to be a Christian, to have the advantage of His wise guidance in life, to walk with Him, this and no other is the way we must go. The Catholic Church in its ongoing witness to Jesus' Good News, strives to have the same sympathetic attitude in its teaching about sexuality as He did, while remaining true in transmitting His teaching to us in its full truth for our full benefit.

In pondering this fundamental text on human sexuality we note that Jesus goes back to human origins when He says "in the beginning of creation." He refers to both the two creation narratives in *Genesis*, the Priestly account in Chapter 1 by quoting the phrase, "God made them male and female" (1:27), and the Yahwist account of Chapter 2 by quoting the phrase "The two shall become one flesh" (2:24). Thus it is an error to try to play off one of these accounts against another, as some do, by preferring the supposedly older Yahwist narrative that emphasizes the unitive meaning of marriage to the Priestly narrative that emphasizes its procreative purpose. The ultimate editor of *Genesis* (whose work, whatever sources he may have used, alone has the Church's guarantee of Divine inspiration) evidently included both accounts with their different emphases so they might complement each other, just as Jesus quotes them together.

Thus we can see that God made us sexual for two reasons. First, the Yahwist account teaches us that human sexuality is for the faithful union of male and female, who are complementary to each other, a union which is not only physical, but psychological and spiritual. *Ephesians* (5:21–32) tells us that this complementary union of love is like that of Christ's own love for His people.[1] Second, the account of *Genesis* 1 teaches us that the second and specifying purpose of human sexuality, essential to us as social beings, is to produce the family on which all human society is built: "Be fertile, multiply, and fill the earth and subdue it" (1:28).

What, then, of a third purpose, obvious enough, and for many of our contemporaries the most important of all: sexual pleasure, "good sex"? To be assured that the Bible does not condemn sexual pleasure one has only to read the *Song of Songs*, "Let my lover come to his garden and eat its choice fruits" (4:16b) and *Qoheleth*, "Enjoy life with the wife you love" (2–9). In the creation story itself Adam cries out with delight on first meeting Eve (*Gen.* 2:21) – evidently anticipating erotic fulfillment.

Yet as Aristotle and St. Thomas Aquinas said, physical pleasure is not an end itself, but a facilitator of good activities. Thus we ought not to eat simply for the pleasure, but because the pleasure of eating both nourishes us and contributes to human conviviality. When physical pleasure becomes an end in itself we are on the road to addiction, since the lust for such pleasure is limitless and uncontrolled, and can only end in self-destruction. Sexual pleasure, therefore, is morally good when it promotes and is controlled by the two essential purposes of sex, the love of man and wife and the building of their family. When it serves these two purposes and is moderated by them without shame it should be profoundly, richly enjoyed. When it is separated from these two purposes it becomes addictive and depersonalizing.

But what is the relation between these two basic purposes for which God created us sexual? Vatican II and the subsequent popes have only declared them to be "inseparable." Prior to Vatican II, Church documents gave priority to the procreative end of marriage and seemed to treat its unitive end as secondary, thus seeming to indicate that it was only a means to procreation. Since love is the highest Gospel value, however, theologians early in the twentieth century began to ask how covenanted married love, the Biblical metaphor for God's own love for us, can be subordinated to any other goal, even the survival of the species. Hence recent Church documents do not compare the two values of marriage but speak of them as coequal, interrelated, and inseparable.

Why are they inseparable? Love is the generic character of all human relationships, which in the sexual relationship is specified by its inseparable linkage to the service of society and human survival by reproduction. Thus the grounds for the Church's insistence that these two purposes are coequal but inseparable is that without one being subordinate to the other, they mutually specify each other. It also follows, contrary to the bias of our present culture, that sexual relationships cannot be merely private affairs between consenting adults, but require the marriage covenant as a social institution necessary to the common good and demanding the community's support.

This seems also to be the sense of the remarkable teaching of John Paul II that our bodies have a "nuptial meaning" because gender differences manifest a specifically human need for a profound, intimate relationship involving the whole person, soul and body. Moreover, this intimate marital relationship grounds all other human relationships – the relationship of parents to children and children to parents, and through the family the relation of friendship to others, and finally our relationships as members of an ever-widening community. In other words, the family built on the unitive love of a man and woman and fruitful in the transmission of human life, is the school of love in which all other human relationships of love are learned. It is not surprising, therefore, that if a family is not sexually whole it may not be able to transmit sexual wholeness to the next generation.

Heterosexuality and Homosexuality

In view of what God in the Bible has told us about why the Creator made us sexual, in judging the morality of any particular use of sexuality we must ask whether it can serve this purpose or whether it is contradictory to it. The first conclusion, which today is very counter-cultural, is that all forms of autoeroticism and extra-marital sex are incompatible with the intrinsic character of our sexuality. Far from it being natural for us to seek sexual pleasure outside of marriage, it is a denial of our true selves. Not only is autoerotic activity sterile, it lacks the unitive relationship with another person. Of course it is not wrong to love ourselves, including our own bodies. St. Paul in speaking of a man's love for his wife actually says in the text already referred to,

> Husbands should love their wives as their own bodies. He who loves his wife loves himself. For no one hates his own body but rather nourishes and cherishes it, even as Christ does the Church, for we are members of His body. (*Eph* 5: 28–29)

But if we love our bodies rightly, to masturbate is indeed self-abuse and its usual consequence is an addiction to merely physical pleasure that will condition the self-abuser to seek mere physical satisfaction, even in intercourse with another. It resembles the addiction to alcohol and drugs that may help a person "relax" or console them in depression, but it ultimately isolates them from genuinely personal relationships.

Jesus' teaching on the purpose of sexuality also excludes extra-marital sex of any kind. If this genital activity outside mar-

Rev. Benedict Ashley, O.P.

riage is merely a search for physical satisfaction as in prostitution or casual sex without a relationship of love, it obviously fails to satisfy our genuine sexual needs. Jesus' teaching on divorce also implies that outside of marriage sexual abstinence is required of all his disciples. The euphemistic New American Bible translation "incapable of marriage" is in the original "eunuch," a strong term used by Jesus, probably to remove any doubt his hearers might have that he meant total sexual abstinence. Before marriage and after the death of one's married partner every Christian is required to abstain from all genital activity.

But why does this apply to extramarital sex between people who truly love each other? This raises the question of what "love" means. Christian "love" has a quite specific meaning. "Love" (*agape*) is not merely to be attracted to another or take pleasure in another, but it is to seek the true good of another. Those who are not permanently committed to each other in marriage and who have sexual relationships cannot honestly say that they love each other in this full sense. If they did they would hasten to marry. And if they could not marry soon, they would wait to have a sexual relationship until they could. The fact that they do not marry means that their love is merely conditional, not unconditional, as true concern for the good of another must be. The conditionality of extra-marital sex always puts the other person at risk. The woman especially is not free from a very real risk of pregnancy unless she is sterilized and abandons hope of children. This risk of begetting a child outside wedlock is also a grave threat to the unwed father who will then have a life-long obligation to his child. Today he may be unable to prevent the woman from killing his child by an abortion. Above all it is a grave injustice to the child to be born illegitimate.

Furthermore, cohabitation without marriage often results in heart-break for that partner who truly desires real self-commitment to the other, but ultimately finds that the other was not so sincerely committed. Of course this often happens in marriage, but at least in marriage the commitment is formal and explicit and sanctioned by society. Thus, extra-marital love can be deeply pas-

80

sionate and a lover can think that he or she intends the good of the other, but for all the intensity of this feeling it is an injustice harmful to the other and to oneself and perhaps to a third party, the child. It cannot be true love as Jesus taught us to love by His unconditional love for us.

If we accept this teaching of Jesus and of the Bible as a whole, then it also becomes clear why genital activity between persons of the same sex is irreconcilable with that teaching. Homosexuals may love each other passionately and with some real concern for the other, but their genital activity is not marital activity. It is not married love, first of all because it cannot produce a family. That this is an essential defect of same-sex love has been shown lately by the efforts of many homosexual couples, especially lesbian couples, to adopt children, or for a lesbian to resort to artificial insemination. The serious question to be raised about such artificial families is whether they are formed primarily in view of the child's good or rather for the good of the same-sex couple. God provided the natural family in which the child is linked to the parents both biologically and by reason of their committed love and sexual complementarity. Children adopted even in a regular marriage often suffer serious difficulties, as is evidenced by the cases frequently reported in the media of their anxious search for their biological parents. It is, of course, better for them to be adopted than to remain orphaned. Yet children adopted or artificially produced by same-sex couples suffer the further deprivation that they do not have the environment provided by the complementarity of father and mother designed by the Creator. Is it not to be feared, therefore, that what really motivates these efforts by same-sex couples to have children, is not the child's good, but a vain effort to justify their relationship?

What then of homosexual relationships considered simply as intimate unions? Can they be reconciled to Jesus' teaching on sexuality? Certainly not if they are promiscuous or casual couplings anymore than promiscuous or casual heterosexual relations can be reconciled with His teaching. Such relations have no genuine element of love but only physical satisfaction and cannot be

Christian. In fact to call them a "relationship" is simply dishonest. Like masturbation, they are merely a form of loving one's own body and trying to get as much pleasure as possible out of it by contact with another body, not a unitive relationship of person to person.

Tragically, through the recent public acceptance of homosexual behavior, a "gay lifestyle" has been fostered in communities where promiscuity is cultivated even more recklessly than is illicit heterosexual behavior in society at large. Though restricted by the AIDS epidemic, this lifestyle may well again flourish if and when this plague comes under control. While it must be granted that promiscuity may, like pedophilia, be compulsive and thus indicate diminished moral responsibility, it would be an insult to deny such responsibility to most homosexuals. Their sexual drives are no more an excuse for a lack of moral self-control than those of heterosexuals.

Some well-intentioned priests and others who minister to homosexuals have concluded, therefore, that the only ethical solution for the gay or lesbian is to seek a stable same-sex partnership that approximates marriage and which is the best that a homosexual can hope to achieve. To facilitate this solution it is even urged by some that society recognize these unions as "marriages" having a legal and social support such as that given to the mutual commitment of married couples. Some who grant that homosexuality is objectively a disorder, argue that nevertheless it is within the natural law. Did not St. Thomas Aquinas consider that in our fallen world polygamy, war, and slavery are within the natural law?[2] They advocate a "theology of compromise" which justifies active homosexuality as the only sexual fulfillment possible for those so oriented. Still other theologians adopt a moral theory according to which morality is determined simply by the proportionate weight of positive and negative values involved in an act and argue that in such homosexual quasi-marriages the positive may outweigh the negative. Finally, some would simply permit it as a lesser evil than promiscuity.

John Paul II in his encyclical *The Splendor of Truth* has shown that these theories of moral reasoning cannot be squared with the

Scriptures, Sacred Tradition, or reason. Some actions, forced sex for example, are clearly intrinsically wrong and cannot be morally justified by circumstances or mere good intentions. An action is "intrinsically immoral" if it is contradictory to the human needs and purposes built into our nature by God. Since, as I have already argued, homosexual activity is contradictory to these needs or purposes, it is intrinsically unethical. The fact that both parties consent does not make what they consent to morally good if in fact it is intrinsically evil and harmful to both. The drug seller and the drug user consent to a transaction that harms both. Consenting adults who engage in homosexual acts are harming the moral as well as the physical integrity of both themselves and their partners.

Some have even argued, "God made me gay, so He must want me to live as a gay." But it is false that God made anyone homosexual anymore than God made some persons blind, deaf, or bald. An adequate theological answer to the problem of evil does not blame the Creator for human suffering, especially for the suffering of the innocent. In our fallen state we are all born into a world distorted by a sinful human history that has deprived every child of the perfect natural familial and social environment which the Creator intended. That a child has been hindered in her or his normal development to heterosexuality whether by genetic defect or defective education and formation is not God's fault, but is due to the misuse by our ancestors and ourselves of God's gifts to us of intelligence and freedom.[3]

That is why the Church can speak of homosexual tendencies as a "disorder," which is suffered by a person who is, perhaps often, not a willing cause of this defect but who ought to recognize it as a defect like any other human defect. We must all deal with our many defects – physical, psychological, and moral – first of all by acknowledging that they are defects. Homosexuals cannot do this by just "coming out." To "come out" is usually nothing but a search for a group that will support the homosexual's denial and rationalizing. The real remedy is for the homosexual to face the hard fact that he or she is not normally heterosexual and must seek a way to become so, or, if this impossible, to live with this defect chastely as we must all do with our sexuality whatever difficulties it may cause for us in the circumstances of our lives. Denial of the facts or self-pity because of them insults human dignity.

Granted that homosexuality is a disorder, what is its cause? As the Vatican has recently said, this remains unknown and it is very probable that it is a symptom not of one but many conditions. Even heterosexuality is probably not simply a genetic given, but requires complex learning for which a healthy family environment is propitious, if not absolutely necessary.

Whether or not a genetic disposition to homosexuality exists, a homosexual orientation can come about through accidents of early psychosexual development or even through later experiences, just as can other forms of erotic fixation.

If we do not fully understand the causes of homosexuality how can we say, as gay activists usually do, that homosexual orientation is always determined early, and is irreversible?[4]

There certainly are cases of persons, like the famous economist John Meynard Keynes, who, after years of enthusiastic homosexual activity, settled down to a happy heterosexual marriage. In fact research seems to have shown that between complete homosexuality and complete heterosexuality there is a range of bisexuality.[5] Thus, young persons who wonder if they are homosexual or who have experimented with gay activity, ought to seek psychological and spiritual diagnosis before stereotyping themselves as gay. Moreover, gay activists ought to seriously consider their responsibility to promote research on the prevention and cure of their difficult condition, as so many with other disabilities have done, rather than to discourage such research on the grounds that it stigmatizes a hopeless limitation.

But let us consider the worst scenario: how shall persons of homosexual orientation who are sure that this is their permanent and irremediable situation, live a happy life? We return to the words of Jesus Himself, "Some are incapable of marriage because they were born so; some, because they were made so by others; some because they have renounced marriage for the sake of the Kingdom of Heaven. Whoever can accept this ought to accept it."

Those who have "renounced marriage for the sake of the Kingdom of Heaven" have accepted St. Paul's recommendation that they, like Mary, Jesus, and Paul freely choose to renounce all genital pleasure:

> I tell you, brothers, the time is running out. From now on, let those having wives act as not having them, those weeping as not weeping, those rejoicing as not rejoicing, those buying as not owning, those using the world as not using it fully. For the world in its present form is passing away. I should like you to be free of anxieties. An unmarried man is anxious about the things of the Lord, how he may please the Lord. But a married man is anxious about the things of the world, how he may please his wife, and he is divided.
>
> An unmarried woman or a virgin is anxious about the things of the Lord, so that she may be holy in both body and spirit. A married woman, on the other hand, is anxious about the things of the world, how she may please her husband. I am telling you this for own benefit, not to impose a restraint up you, but for the sake of propriety and adherence to the Lord without distraction. (I *Cor* 7: 29–35).

Thus, the attitude of the Christian Church, following the words and example of Jesus Himself, is just the reverse of the attitude of those theologians who excuse homosexual behavior on the ground of compromise with our fallen condition. God made us all in the beginning to marry happily, and this is still the call of most Christians. In our fallen world, however, the married have to struggle to prevent the problems of domestic life from so absorbing their energies that they forget their ultimate goal as Christians. When the Pharisees asked Jesus about what would happen in heaven to the widow who had lost seven husbands, He answered with, I imagine, an amused smile on his lips, "You are misled because you do not know the scriptures or the power of God. At the resurrection they neither marry nor are given in marriage but are like the angels in heaven." (*Mt* 22:29–30, attested also in *Mk* 12:23–25 and *Lk* 20:34–36).

While God does not cause evil, he always brings a greater good out of the evil his creatures have caused. The homosexual condition, therefore, can become the occasion of a great good, namely a celibate life lived for the glory of God, freed of domesticity and devoted single-mindedly to building God's Kingdom. In such a life the spiritual fatherhood and spiritual motherhood of married life can still be attained and are even facilitated. This is why the Catholic Church, in spite of declining priestly vocations, still requires celibacy for priests. Celibacy undertaken in view of the Kingdom is a liberating condition, not an onerous one, and to it especially applies Jesus' saying, "My yoke is easy and my burden light."

As Jesus and St. Paul indicate, to freely choose celibacy when one could marry, or to accept it willingly when one is not yet married, or can never marry, is not just for those in the ordained clergy or those in religious communities. It may be the call of God to any Christian, and some are called by the very fact that they cannot marry. They can be confident that the grace to fulfill this vocation will not be denied them. This is the case with the person with a fixed homosexual orientation. The very fact that one is not suited for marriage is a call from God to live a celibate life and to make celibacy a way of liberation. Every vocation in life is difficult, a way of the Cross for both married and unmarried, but by the grace of God it can be lived well and happily. We may sometimes fail in our vocation, but the mercy of God will put us back on the road and bring us safely home. Therefore, the homosexual who has come to understand that this is his or her vocation in life – a cross to carry, but a liberating opportunity – will not yield to self-pity, but will face the truth and live by it.

As for heterosexuals and especially the married, the courage of chaste homosexuals should kindle not pity but admiration, and a determination to give them every support possible including every social and legal defense against violence or unjust discrimination. For those gays and lesbians who have not yet found it possible to accept this call from Jesus, we should show the riches of our sympathy and prayers. We should help them have courage not to despair or to lapse into a reckless gay or lesbian ways of life, and for those who mistakenly hope for a kind of permanent same-sex relationship we should pray that they come to see that it can be transformed into a chaste friendship free of the contradictions of genital activity. Finally, from those who are striving to follow the virginal Christ the unmarried should learn chastity for themselves and the married should recognize the splendor of a love that can transcend this world.

Endnotes

1. Some important exegetes, such as Barth and Westermann, even claim that the text of *Genesis* 1:27. "God created a human in his image, in the divine image he created this human, male and female he created them" indicates that the image of God is found not in male or female individually, at least not perfectly, but in their complementarity.

2. Aquinas (see *Summa Theologiae* 1-II q. 100 ad 3) included war and slavery within the scope of natural law as a punishment for the sin of fighting an unjust war and similarly slavery. The polygymy of the Old Testament he considered a divine dispensation from a secondary principle of the natural law for the survival of the Chosen People, *S. Th.*, II-II q. 154, a. 2 ad 2; Suppl. q.65, a.5, ad 2. It is difficult to see how he could have accepted any such reason to justify homosexuality which he considered contrary to the male-female relationship which for him is paradigmatically "natural" *S.Th.* II-II, qq. 11-12.

3. "Original sin" is best understood as our "sinful origin," i.e., the effects on us of the sins of all human history beginning with our first parents. A child is not born a sinner, as some suppose the Church to teach, but the victim of the sins of the human race into which he or she is born. The child is victimized first of all by being deprived of the grace God intended the child to receive from his or her parents and then from all the distortions of God's good creation caused by human sin. A child becomes a sinner him- or herself only when he or she knowingly and freely accepts the world's sinful ways.

4. Gay activists continue to assert with only anecdotal evidence that sexual orientation is irreversible and that the claims of some clinicians to have enabled homosexuals to enter into satisfactory hetero-

Rev. Benedict Ashley, O.P.

sexual marriages are spurious. My arguments in no way depend on claims of either side in this debate, which can only be settled by scientifically valid research to which neither claim has yet been adequately subjected. It is notoriously difficult to measure the success of psychological therapy. What is indefensible, however, is the claim of gay propaganda that the removal by the American Psychiatric Association of homosexuality as a psychological disorder from its manual is proof that the psychiatric profession has discovered that sexual orientation is irreversible after early childhood. It is well-known that this decision was not based on any rigorous research, but was the result of political activity of a group within the Association who argued that the inclusion of this category in the manual stigmatized gays.

5. On this topic see Beth A. Firestein, ed., *Bisexuality: The Psychology and Politics of an Invisible Minority* (Thousand Oaks, CA: Sage Publications, 1996). The research surveyed in these essays show that various degrees of bisexuality are often lumped together as homosexuality. Some contributors complain that bisexuals are even more socially oppressed than homosexuals!

"An Intrinsically Disordered Inclination"
John Finnis

What the Church teaches about homosexual inclinations

The Church "refuses to consider the person as a 'heterosexual' or a 'homosexual' and insists that every person has a fundamental identity: the creature of God and, by grace, his child and heir to eternal life."[1] Each person also has a "sexual identity": either male or female, man or woman.[2] The Church does not use the term "sexual identity" as some people do, who claim that people have "sexual identities" as homosexuals, heterosexuals, bisexuals, pedophiles, and so forth. Instead, the Church teaches that each male should accept his sexual identity as a man, and each female her sexual identity as a woman; and that means accepting that one is *different* from and *complementary to*[3] – and equal in dignity with[4] – persons of the opposite sex (gender).

The Church has sometimes spoken of "homosexual persons." Anyone who has a "more or less strong tendency towards" sexual activity with a person or persons of the same sex can be so described. Of course, as is well known, most such persons are *also* "heterosexual persons." That is to say, most people who engage, or have an inclination to engage, in homosexual activity also engage, or are more or less inclined to engage, in sexual activity with a person or persons of the opposite sex. Very many homosexual persons – persons with homosexual inclinations – marry and have children by their spouse. Not all do, and there are some, relatively quite few, who have a sexual urge but lack the psychophysical capacity for marital intercourse.

The Church observes that in some homosexual persons the homosexual inclination (= orientation) comes, it seems, "from a false education, from a lack of normal sexual development, from habit, from bad example, or from other similar causes, and is transitory or at least not incurable."[5] But the Church also observes that "the number of men and women who have *deep-seated* homosexual tendencies is not negligible,"[6] and that some homosexual persons may be "definitively such because of some kind of innate instinct or a pathological constitution judged to be incurable."[7] Acknowledging the last-mentioned class of persons, the Church is well aware of people who "conclude that their tendency is so natural that it justifies in their case homosexual relations within a sincere communion of life and love analogous to marriage, insofar as such homosexuals feel incapable of enduring a solitary life."[8]

But the Church, today as always, rejects that way of arguing from "nature." The Christian teaching, from the outset, has been that no homosexual acts are ever justified, even the acts of someone whose inclination to engage in them is "innate" (that is, present at birth) and, in one sense of the word, "natural." Accordingly, the Church's *Catechism* reaffirms that every such inclination, whether innate or pathological, incurable or curable, permanent or transitory, is an *objective disorder*,[9] an *intrinsically disordered* inclination.[10]

The reason why even the most deep-seated homosexual tendency must be called disordered is straightforward. Every such tendency, inclination or orientation[11] "is a more or less strong tendency ordered toward an intrinsic moral evil."[12] Of course, "the particular *inclination* of the homosexual person is not a sin"[13] – for a sin is committed only in a choice. But the inclination is precisely an *inclination to choose* a homosexual act – a sex act with a person of the same sex. And, like every other kind of non-marital sex act, any and every homosexual *act* is a seriously disordered kind of activity which, if freely and deliberately chosen, is a serious sin. An inclination which one cannot choose to pursue without serious moral evil is obviously a disordered inclination. So: "the particular inclination of the homosexual person . . . is a more or less strong tendency ordered [i.e., directed] toward an intrinsic moral evil, *and thus* the inclination itself must be seen as *an objective dis - order.*"[14] The definitive edition of the *Catechism of the Catholic Church* first points out that homosexual *acts* are always "intrinsically disordered" (§ 2357) and then goes on, in the following paragraph, to describe the *inclination* in precisely the same terms: "intrinsically disordered."

Why the Church's teaching about homosexual inclinations is right

The Church's teaching about homosexual inclinations is made with full awareness of modern psychological and biological research into the origins of these inclinations. But it does not rely on the judgment of those researchers who are convinced that homosexuality is a "psychiatric disorder." Nor does is it contradicted or challenged or unsettled by the opinion of those who hold that it is *not* a psychiatric disorder. The Church's teaching about these inclinations rests instead on the Catholic doctrine about the *choice* to engage in homosexual *acts*. This is a *moral* doctrine, a teaching about what is right (or wrong), good (or worthless and harmful), and choiceworthy (or sinful).

From its earliest years, the Church has understood its moral doctrine as not only a matter of faith but also fully in line with human *nature*. St. Paul teaches clearly about this in his letter to the Romans (*Rom.* 2: 14–15). But Jesus has already made the point by his profound teachings on human sexual identity (*Matt.* 19: 4), and on the marital communion of man and woman which, on the basis of that complementarity of identities, was established *"from the beginning"* (i.e., in the intentions of God the creator of nature) (*Matt.* 19: 8). As Jesus makes clear, this natural communion requires for its integrity not only the sexual intercourse of the spouses (*Matt.* 19: 5), but also the complete and unwavering mastery and overcoming – by everyone, married or unmarried – of every desire for sexual contact or enjoyment outside marriage (*Matt.* 5: 27). To look on anyone with lust is "adultery," that is, an offense – even by the unmarried – *against marriage*, a relationship both profoundly natural and sustainable only by *moral* aspiration. I shall show, below, why this must be so.

Some of the greatest theologians and philosophers have explained the relationship between human nature, the natural world as a whole, and the truths of morality. Morality concerns, not what simply is or is deep-seated or usual, but rather the *good*, and the various kinds of good (*goods*), which *should be* sought, chosen, and done. Everything that should be, and is choiceworthy, is natural and grounded in the givens of human nature. But not everything we find in our nature is a pointer to what is good, choiceworthy, and reasonable. For example, as St. Thomas Aquinas, the master theorist of natural law morality, points out, we all have "a *natural inclination* to follow our bodily feelings and desires even against the good of being reasonable."[15] This is one of many "natural" – i.e., innate, deep-seated, typical – inclinations which should *not* simply be followed! Others are found more in some people's nature than in others': some people are more inclined to anger, including immoral anger, than others, some are more inclined to greed, some to crippling fear, and so forth. So, as John Paul II teaches, "natural inclinations take on moral relevance only insofar as they refer to the human person and the person's *authentic fulfillment* . . ."[16] Aquinas, following a lead from Aristotle's research and reflections, reminds his readers that homosexual inclinations – e.g., the desire of some men to have sex with other men – arise in some cases from pleasure-seeking which has initiated and sustained a corrupt taste for this sort of behavior, a bad habit, but in other cases from a defective psycho-physical constitution (i.e., from inclinations incipiently present even from conception). The way these inclinations originate in a particular person does not affect the fact that, just insofar as they incline that person towards sex acts with persons of the same sex, they incline not towards but away from authentic fulfillment.

Human fulfillment consists in the actualizing, in the lives of persons and their communities, those basic human goods towards which the first principles of practical reason – the very foundations of conscience – direct us.[17] Among these basic human goods is the *good of marriage*.[18] The Church often speaks of the goods of marriage: (1) loving friendship between wife and husband, and (2) procreating and educating any children who may be conceived from the spouses marital intercourse.[19] They are interdependent goods: this is a friendship sealed by a commitment to exclusiveness and permanence, a commitment of a kind made appropriate by marriage's orientation to the procreation and education of the children of the husband/father and wife/mother; and that raising of children is most appropriately undertaken as a long-term, even lifelong commitment of the spouse-parents. Being interdependent, these goods can also be properly described as two aspects of a single basic human good, the good of marriage itself. In the Church's most explicit teaching on the foundations of its moral doctrine, in which Pope John Paul points to the basic human goods as the first principles of the natural moral law, this single though basic good is called: "the communion of persons in marriage."[20]

The whole Christian teaching on sex has, from the beginning, done no more, and no less, than point out the ways in which *every* kind of sex act other than authentic marital intercourse is opposed to the good of marriage. The more distant a kind of sex act is from the marital kind, the more seriously disordered and, in itself, immoral it is.

How do non-marital sex acts oppose the good of marriage? The next few paragraphs sketch one kind of answer to that question. It is only one of many ways in which the question has been answered. It is suggested by one of Aquinas's central teachings about the morality of marital intercourse, an often misunderstood, but important and true teaching which the Church itself also upholds.

In Christian marriage the personality, individuality, and equality of the spouses is fully respected. The marital communion is not a submerging of the two persons into one. But it is a communion, a bringing-together of their wills in their mutual commitment; of their wills and minds in shared understanding and faith and hope; of their wills, minds, and feelings in shared joys, cares, and sadnesses; and of their wills, minds, feelings, and bodies in sexual intercourse. That intercourse, when it is truly marital, enables them to experience and actualize their mutual commitment and communion at all levels of their being: biological, emotional, rational, and volitional. It is only truly marital when it has the characteristics of the two-sided good of marriage itself: friendship and openness to procreation. A sexual act is marital only when (1) it is an act of the generative *kind*, that is, culminates in a union of the generative organs in which the wife accepts into her genital tract her husband's genital organ and the seed he thereby gives her; and (2) it is an act of friendship in which each is seeking to express affection for and commitment to, and the desire to benefit and give pleasure to, and share pleasure with, the other spouse as the very person to whom he or she is committed in marriage. These two conditions are also inter-linked: only an act of the generative kind (in the sense just specified) truly *unites* the spouses at all levels, biologically as well as at the level of feelings and intentions – and such an act does so even if, at the time of intercourse, they cannot in fact generate.

So a married couple's sexual act is not truly marital if, for example, one or both of the spouses is wishing he or she were doing this with someone else, or is imagining doing so, or is willing to engage in this activity with any attractive person who could bring him or her to orgasmic release. Think of someone whose frame of mind is: I am willing to do this with some other attractive person, but the only available person at present is my spouse, so I'll do it with her/him. Such a person is disabled by that frame of mind from making and carrying through a truly marital choice to engage in intercourse. In the technical phrase of the theologians, this person is engaging in intercourse *for pleasure alone*. His or her act of intercourse is depersonalized, not an act of marital friendship. That is why the Church teaches[21] that such a choice is always morally flawed; and in some kinds of instance it is a serious sin against the integrity and authenticity of marriage and marital life.[22]

The good of marriage is an intrinsic good, not a mere means to any other end. But it is also true that the well-being of children greatly depends upon the marital commitment of their parents. That commitment tends to be strengthened by marital intercourse which respects the integrity and authenticity – the purity – of their marriage. And it is weakened at its heart by intercourse which is not truly marital , but rather expressive of self-indulgence. So anyone who thinks clearly, has the well-being of children at heart, and recognizes the good of marital communion, will judge wrong- ful every kind of sex act which is not truly marital.

One reason for that moral judgment is this. One cannot engage in truly marital intercourse if one is willing, even conditionally willing, to engage – i.e., is not set against engaging, in some pos- sible circumstances – in this sort of behavior (deliberate sexual stimulation towards orgasm) outside marriage or in one or other of the non-marital ways. Such a willingness, unless and until one reverses it by repenting of it, so deforms one's will that one is dis- abled from engaging in a free, rational, sentient, and bodily act which would *really* express, actualize, foster, and enable one's spouse to experience the good of marriage and of one's own com- mitment (self-giving) in marriage. Of course, one may be under the illusion that one's act, though performed with this divided, impure willingness, is still an expression and experiencing of the good of marriage. But this can be no more than an illusion, which rational reflection punctures. And a spouse who knows or senses that the other spouse *is willing* – even conditionally or hypotheti- cally – to do this kind of thing outside (before, during, or after) marriage is likely to experience the act as not an expression and actualization of *marital* commitment. That is why such a willing- ness saps marriage at its core. [23]

So: nobody who is or wishes to be a spouse, and no one who considers it reasonable for people to become spouses, can judge it reasonable for human beings to seek sexual satisfaction in an extra-marital way. For approval of extra-marital sex acts, even of other people's acts or of the sex acts of people who could never marry, has two implications. (1) It implies that anyone and every- one *should* approve of such acts, i.e., should regard them as kinds of act not excluded by reasonableness. And (2) it is a form of conditional willingness to engage in such acts. Therefore, it entails (necessarily implies) also (3) that married couples, spouses, should approve of and be conditionally willing to perform non-marital acts. But such a conclusion is directly opposed to the good of marriage, of the spouses as committed friends, and of any children who may have resulted from their marital union and be dependent upon the purity which is near the heart of its stability.

Homosexual sex acts, even between people who could never consummate a marriage, or between people who wish, at the time, to be committed to each other in a lifelong friendship, can never be marital. To judge them morally acceptable is opposed to the good of marriage, a basic human good. So they cannot be regarded as morally acceptable.

The relationship of same-sex couples can never be marriage. The easiest way to see this is to ask oneself why same-sex sex acts should be restricted to couples rather than three-somes, four-somes, etc., or rather than couples or other groups whose membership rotates at agreed intervals. Nothing in the gay ideology can, or even seriously tries, to explain or defend the exclusiveness or permanence of same-sex partnerships or their limitation to couples. The practice and experience of homosexual relationships is dramatic confirmation that, once one departs from the institution of *marriage* as a committed, exclusive, and permanent sexual relationship between a woman and a man, there are no solid grounds for making one's sexual relationships even *imitate* real marriage.[24]

A final word on "sexual orientation"

The shifty phrase "sexual orientation" is an important obstacle to clear thinking. It spreads darkness over the law and popular discussions by hiding the distinction between emotional inclinations, dispositions, or interests and actual or conditional *willing - ness*. Willingness is, or results from, a choice – perhaps a conditional choice ("I am willing to do this if I find someone attractive and a safe opportunity . . ."), perhaps an unconditional and immediate choice. Emotional inclinations, dispositions, and interests, on the other hand, do not engage one's moral responsibility unless they result from earlier choices or are allowed to lead one to such a choice.

> The phrase "sexual orientation" is radically equivocal. Particularly as used by promoters of "gay rights," the phrase ambiguously assimilates two things which that [the law] hitherto has carefully distinguished: (I) a psychological or psychosomatic disposition inwardly orienting one *towards* homosexual activity; (II) the deliberate decision so to orient one's public *behavior* as to express or *manifest* one's active interest in and endorsement of homosexual *conduct* and/or forms of life which presumptively involve such conduct. . . . laws or proposed laws outlawing "discrimination based on sexual orientation" are always interpreted by "gay rights" movements as going far beyond discrimination based merely on A's belief that B is sexually attracted to persons of the same sex. Instead (it is observed), "gay rights" movements interpret the phrase as extending full legal protection to *public* activities intended specifically to promote, procure and facilitate homosexual *conduct*.[25]

St. Paul's reflections on homosexual vice, in *Romans* 1: 19–28, makes it clear that what matters is not inclinations but the will (the debased *mind*) and chosen conduct. With minds darkened, "women exchanged natural intercourse for unnatural, and in the same way men . . . committed shameless acts with men . . ." (*Rom.* 2: 21, 26–28).

And it is important to be clear that the natural intercourse wrongly set aside by people who fail to allow reason to master their inclinations is not simply heterosexual. Rather, it is *marital*. That is, it is sexually complementary, and in every sexual act is expressive – physically, emotionally, and intellectually – of both the essential marital goods: procreation, and a friendship which is exclusive and permanently committed.

Endnotes

1. Congregation for the Doctrine of the Faith, *Letter to the Bishops of the Catholic Church on the Pastoral Care of Homosexual Persons*, 1 October 1986, sec. 16.

2. *Catechism of the Catholic Church* (revised edition 1997), 2333, 2393.

3. Ibid. 2333, 2393.

4. Ibid. 2334–35, 2393.

5. Sacred Congregation for the Doctrine of the Faith, *Declaration on Certain Questions concerning Sexual Ethics*, 29 December 1975, sec. 8.

6. *Catechism of the Catholic Church* (rev. ed.), 2358.

7. *Declaration on Certain Questions concerning Sexual Ethics*, sec. 8. In the Latin version "some kind of innate" is replaced by *"quasi-innatus,"* which means "as if innate [though not, or not necessarily, innate]." In the first Italian edition of the *Catechism of the Catholic Church*, 2358, the word "deep-seated" in the phrase "deep-seated homosexual tendencies" was rendered "innate," and this was changed in the revision of 1997 because, as Cardinal Ratzinger explained, competent experts consider that it has not been proven that homosexual tendencies are ever present from conception. But actually nothing of moral importance turns on whether "innate" or "quasi-innate" or "deep-seated" is used in this context: see text at notes 15 and 16 below.

8. Ibid.

9. *Pastoral Care of Homosexual Persons*, sec. 3.

10. *Catechism of the Catholic Church* (rev. ed.), 2358.

11. The Church's documents on the matter treat all these words as referring to the same thing.

12. *Pastoral Care of Homosexual Persons*, sec. 3.

13. Ibid.

14. Ibid.

15. See Finnis, *Aquinas* 93.

16. John Paul II, Encyclical Letter *Veritatis Splendor*, 6 August 1993, sec. 50 (emphasis added).

17. See *Veritatis Splendor*, secs. 13, 48 ("the primordial moral requirement of loving and respecting the person as an end and never as a mere means also implies, by its very nature, respect for certain fundamental goods"); 50; also 78, 79.

18. E.g., *Catechism of the Catholic Church,* 2333.

19. Ibid. 2201, 2249.

20. *Veritatis Splendor,* sec. 13. St. Thomas Aquinas long ago identified this as a single though complex primary (basic) human good: see John Finnis, *Aquinas: Moral, Political and Legal Theory* (Oxford University Press, 1998) 82, 143.

21. See decree of the Holy Office against the errors of the laxists, 2 March 1679, no. 9.

22. See Finnis, *Aquinas* 149.

23. This line of thought is explored in depth and detail in Finnis, "The Good of Marriage and the Morality of Sexual Relations: Some Philosophical and Historical Observations," *American Journal of Jurisprudence* 42 (1997) 97 at 119–26. See also pp. 126–34, exploring the reasons why spouses who know that, though they have not tried to prevent conception, they cannot conceive (i.e., are naturally infertile or have become sterile e.g., as a result of age) can nevertheless engage in authentically marital acts of the reproductive *kind*, while same-sex partners cannot engage in acts of the reproductive kind, i.e., in marital intercourse.

24. See ibid., pp. 123–34, especially notes 108, 131–33.

25. John Finnis, "Law, Morality, and 'Sexual Orientation,'" *Notre Dame Law Review* 69 (1994) 1049–76 at 1053–54.

Law

"Life Partners" Legislation
Anthony Cardinal Bevilacqua

Editors' Note: *On April 22, 1998 Anthony Cardinal Bevilacqua testi -*
fied before the Philadelphia City Council in opposition to five bills,
extending to so-called "domestic partners" or "life partners" various
benefits reserved to spouses or to blood relatives. The testimony is print -
ed here with the permission of Cardinal Bevilacqua.

I am here to testify today because of the gravity of these five
bills regarding life partners and domestic partners being considered by Council. I appear before you confident that my position –
the position of the Catholic Church – is grounded in a firm basis
of morality, custom and faith. I am testifying in person so that the
members of the council as well as the public will hear the Catholic
Church's true position on marriage, the traditional family, homosexuality and the proposed life-partners legislation.

In 1996, this Council held hearings on ordinances regarding
so-called *domestic partners*. Today three ordinances refer to *life part -*
ners while two ordinances refer to *domestic partners*. Yet both terms
refer to the same relationship. The nomenclature is different; the
meaning and consequences of the suggested measures are the
same.

The bills before you individually and, more importantly, taken
together attempt to do no less than create a sense of moral, cultural and legal equality between marriage and same-sex partnerships, so-called *life partnerships*. They reflect an attempt to cast
aside marriage as our legal standard and to establish a legitimacy
for homosexual unions as well as heterosexual partnerships outside of marriage. However, the marital relationship shared by husband and wife constitutes the only true and lasting life partnership.

Our position is supported by many religious leaders representing many varied denominations. It is uplifting that one can see and hear these leaders speaking together in one voice. To know that so many religious and community leaders have come together, united on this issue, should not be a surprise to anyone. We have done so before and, if need be, will do so again.

The surprise is not that we have come together, but that we must continue to speak out in favor of marriage and the traditional family in the face of constant assaults on these sacred, time-honored and vital institutions. It is deeply disturbing that every few years we have to come before the City Council to offer testimony in defense of traditional marriage and the family. Perhaps those behind these bills are hoping that we will grow tired or that our message will become outdated or muted. If so, they are grossly mistaken! Though we are of many faiths, we are of one voice.

At the outset I must state unequivocally that the Catholic Church condemns as immoral any act of unjust discrimination against homosexual persons. The Church's teaching on the issue of homosexuals is clearly pronounced in the *Catechism of the Catholic Church*, which states that homosexual people "must be accepted with respect, compassion and sensitivity. Every sign of unjust discrimination in their regard should be avoided" (No. 2358). The Catholic Church clearly teaches that a homosexual orientation in itself in not immoral. Violence and hatred directed at a homosexual person is sinful and wrong.

It is troubling that the issue of life partners has been framed in terms of discrimination. The Archdiocese of Philadelphia works constantly to ensure that our actions and words reflect our firm belief that discrimination against any individual is completely unacceptable. To accuse the Catholic Church of unjust discrimination because it labels homosexual behavior as sinful or because it opposes these bills can only be interpreted as a total disregard for truth and honesty.

We have nothing but loving concern for those who oppose our position, including those who are homosexual. We recognize that all persons are gifts from God and deserving of our love and respect. However, we ask those who disagree with our position to understand that one can love and respect other persons without wanting the government to honor or provide special incentives for their lifestyle.

Some who support these bills allege that their goal is not to equate same-sex life partnerships with marriage, but to avoid discrimination. However, other supporters of these bills concede that their ultimate goal is to establish legal status for so-called *same-sex marriages*. They argue that the definition of marriage has to change with the times. For the Catholic Church, the issue has always been that of preserving and defending the sacred institution of marriage and traditional family life. It has never been a matter of discrimination.

Each year our parish and archdiocesan schools educate over 111,000 students of all races, beliefs and varied incomes. Twenty of our schools are composed solely of minority students, the vast majority of whom are non-Catholic. Each and every student is given the attention and educational assistance he or she needs. We offer this education without discrimination.

Many of you know that the Archdiocese of Philadelphia is the largest private provider of social services in the commonwealth. Each year we serve hundreds of thousands of people of all races, of varied incomes and of all beliefs, even those who profess no religious belief. In response to God's call, we help to clothe the naked, feed the hungry and house the homeless. In addition we provide services to those who suffer with HIV and AIDS. In these humanitarian efforts, all are given assistance without discrimination.

Our human services and educational programs are well-known. However, many people may not know about two archdiocesan programs that go more directly to the issue at hand.

The archdiocese supports a program for Catholics who are homosexual. This program, called *Courage,* assists those who turn to us for help. We offer them love, compassion and support in their desire to live chaste lives. Our faith teaches us that all people are gifts from God. How could we respond otherwise?

Another program, called *Encourage,* is offered for the families of homosexuals. This program provides education, support and love for these family members.

The real issues at hand, marriage and the traditional family, are too important to be lost in the confusion of the debate. These values are too central to all of society. The definition of marriage, the union of a man and a woman, is timeless. Marriage does not change to fit momentary whims or to be "politically correct." Too many people in the media and business worlds already have created an environment where people no longer speak of *husbands and wives.* They talk about *partners.*

I emphatically repeat what I stated five years ago when I testified before the Council, because the truth has not changed and will not change. At that time I testified that such bills are dangerous because they attempt to cast aside marriage as our legal standard of legitimate cohabitation. They intend to give legitimacy to homosexual cohabitation outside of marriage. This is a legitimacy which neither homosexual nor heterosexual cohabitation now enjoys and which, for the common good of the city, should not be given. The legislation communicates to the whole of society, but especially to our youth, that extramarital and homosexual relationships are the natural, moral and legal equivalent of marriage and the family. They endeavor to nullify the fact that committed, traditional marriages and stable families constitute the foundation on which a lasting and civilized society is built.

Marriage and family life have a unique and fundamental role in society. This role springs from the fact that the permanent commitment of husband and wife in marriage is intrinsically tied to the procreation and education of children. This leads eventually to the necessary support of society.

The health and well-being of our city depends on stable families. As elected leaders of our city, you are called to defend the sacred institution of marriage and to support traditional family life. Do not become another negative force in society which gradually erases the term *marriage* from our vocabulary.

Members of the City Council, I submit that the actions of the Catholic Church are based on compassion, justice and equality before God.

One can recognize that each person is a gift from God, yet one does not have to condone every behavior of that person. Therefore, I urge you to reject legislation that gives legal validation to life partners and compels businesses and taxpayers to subsidize these relationships. Just because one's relationship is not validated by law or subsidized by taxpayers does not mean that one is facing unjust discrimination.

A stable civilization needs a stable family life. Therefore, law and public policy should seek to stabilize the traditional family structure through support, protection, enhancement and encouragement. As Archbishop of Philadelphia, shepherd for nearly a half-million Catholics in the city of Philadelphia, and as a citizen of this great city, I respectfully exhort you to reject these bills and to voice your support for marriage and traditional family life.

Members of The City Council, I again extend my hand to you. Together we must work to support the institution of marriage and to strengthen the traditional family. If we are successful, a stronger, healthier Philadelphia and society will surely emerge.

Domestic-Partners Legislation
John Cardinal O'Connor

Editors' note: The following is taken from a homily delivered by Cardinal O'Connor from the pulpit of St. Patrick's Cathedral on May 24, 1998. His Eminence commented on proposed New York City legislation which would have made marital benefits available to unmarried hetero - sexual and homosexual domestic partners registered with the city. The text of the homily first appeared in May 28, 1998, edition of Catholic New York, *and is reprinted here with Cardinal O'Connor's permission.*

As Archbishop of New York, I am asked from time to time by both Catholics and members of other religious faiths, as well as by individuals in public life and in public office, to comment on matters of public policy or to explain Church teaching on such matters. Such is the case regarding the proposed New York City Domestic Partnership Legislation under consideration by the City Council of New York.

It is my understanding that the advocates of this proposed legislation sincerely believe that various individuals in our society are currently being deprived of their due, or that at least certain benefits are not currently guaranteed or protected by law. I can certainly understand such beliefs, while at the same time trying to examine the proposed legislation conscientiously to discern what it actually prescribes and effects, at least in the unamended version available at this time, prior to hearings and the amendment process.

Before presenting those elements of Church teaching that I believe to be most pertinent to the proposed legislation, I think it appropriate to observe that men and women of good will have argued questions of the relative rights of individuals in relation to one another and to society at large from the earliest days of our republic. The same is true about the rights of individuals and the obligations of government. There is nothing new or prejudicial, therefore, in examining proposed domestic partnership legislation from various or differing viewpoints, without questioning sincerity or good faith on the part of all.

The Church expresses its own observations on such matters both because asked to do so and because of its legitimate involvement in so many critical societal activities, including, but not limited to, child care, health care, education, charitable activities and so on. The Church's involvement in such activities is often at the direct request of and on the basis of contracts with government, including the City of New York.

One further observation is critical. The Archdiocese of New York, in keeping with Church teaching, tends to examine all proposed legislation regarding human relationships from the critically important perspective of its potential impact on marriage and family. The press, for example, has generally reported the proposal as legislation to make domestic partners equal to married spouses. Within the frame of reference already provided here, then, the Archdiocese offers the following observation concerning the proposed domestic partnership legislation dominantly from this perspective: What might be reasonably perceived as its potential impact on marriage and family? So, for example, the Holy See's Charter on the Rights of the Family (1983) observes that whereas "[all] persons have the right to the free choice of their state of life and thus to marry and establish a family or to remain single," yet "[t]he institutional value of marriage should be upheld by the public authorities; the situation of nonmarried couples must not be placed on the same level as marriage duly contracted."

In a letter to the world's heads of state dated March 19, 1994, our Holy Father Pope John Paul II stated:

> It is in the family, I believe, that we find a human resource which produces the best creative energies of the social fabric. This is something which every state

ought carefully to safeguard. Without infringing on the autonomy of a reality which they can neither produce nor replace, civil authorities have a duty, in effect, to strive to promote the harmonious growth of the family, not only from the point of view of its social vitality but also from that of its moral and spiritual health. . . .

The leaders of the nations owe it to themselves to reflect deeply and in conscience on this. . . .

An institution as natural, fundamental and universal as the family cannot be manipulated by anyone.

Who could give such a mandate to individuals or institutions? The family is part of the heritage of humanity!

The same Pope stated in a letter to families on February 2, 1994:

Even if someone chooses to remain single, the family continues to be, as it were, his existential horizon, that fundamental community in which the whole network of social relations is grounded, from the closest and most immediate to the most distant. . . .

The family has always been considered as the first and basic expression of man's social nature. . . . The family originates in a marital communion described by the Second Vatican Council as a "covenant," in which man and woman "give themselves to each other and accept each other." . . .

The children born to them – and here is the challenge – should consolidate that covenant, enriching and deepening the conjugal communion of the father and mother. . . . Married couples need to be well aware of this. From the outset they need to have their hearts and thoughts turned toward the God "from whom every family is named" so that their fatherhood and motherhood will draw from that source the power to be continually renewed in love. . . .

In marriage man and woman are so firmly united as to become – to use the words of the *Book of Genesis* – "one flesh" (*Gen.* 2:24). Male and female in the physical constitution, the two human subjects, even though physically different, share equally in the capacity to live "in truth and love." This capacity, characteristic of the human being as a person, has at the same time both a spiritual and a bodily dimension. It is also through the body that man and woman are predisposed to form a "communion of persons" in marriage. When they are united by the conjugal covenant in such a way as to become "one flesh" their union ought to take place "in truth and love," and thus express the maturity proper to persons created in the image and likeness of God.

In his apostolic exhortation in 1981, our Holy Father, Pope John Paul II, observed: "'Since the Creator of all things has established the conjugal partnership as the beginning and basis of human society,' the family is 'the first and vital cell of society.'"

He goes on to say:

The family has vital and organic links with society, since it is its foundation and nourishes it continually through its role of service to life: It is from the family that citizens come to birth, and it is within the family that they find the first school of the social virtues that are the animating principle of the existence and development of society itself. . . .

Just as the intimate connection between the family and society demands that the family be open to and participate in society and its development, so also it requires that society should never fail in its fundamental task of respecting and fostering the family.

The family and society have complementary functions in defending and fostering the good of each and every human being. But society – more specifically the state – must recognize that "the family is a society in its own original right." . . .

In the conviction that the good of the family is an indispensable and essential value of the civil community, the public authorities must do everything possible to ensure that families have all those aids – economic, social, educational, political and cultural assistance – that they need in order to face all their responsibilities in a human way.

In its Charter of the Rights of the Family, the Holy See asserts, among other principles, the following:

– The family is based on marriage, that intimate union of life in complementarity between a man and a woman which is constituted in the freely contracted and publicly expressed indissoluble bond of matrimony and is open to the transmission of life. . . .

– The family, a natural society, exists prior to the state or any other community and possesses inherent rights which are inalienable.

– The family constitutes, much more than a mere juridical, social and economic unit, a community of love and solidarity which is uniquely suited to teach and transmit cultural, ethical, social, spiritual and religious values essential for the development and well-being of its own members and of society. . . .

– The experience of different cultures throughout history has shown the need for society to recognize and defend the institution of the family.

– Society, and in a particular manner the state and international organizations, must protect the family through measures of a political, economic, social and juridical character, which aim at consolidating the unity and stability of the family so that it can exercise its specific function.

– The rights, the fundamental needs, the well-being and the values of the family, even though they are progressively safeguarded in some cases, are often ignored and not rarely undermined by laws, institutions and socio-economic programs. . . .

– The Catholic Church, aware that the good of the person, of society and of the Church herself passes by way of the family, has always held it part of her mission to proclaim to all the plan of God instilled in human nature concerning marriage and the family, to promote these two institutions and to defend them against all those who attack them.

That these teachings and positions are in no way unique to the Catholic Church needs little verification. Jewish and Christian scholars of the ages have articulated similar and generally identical convictions, namely that the lifelong commitment of one man to one woman in marriage gives full expression to the kind of relationship which is best suited to the procreation, rearing and education of children. Moreover, legislators and courts in our land have ratified and been guided by such convictions from time immemorial. So, for example, more than a century ago in *Maynard vs. Hill*, the U.S. Supreme Court declared that marriage "is an institution, in the maintenance of which, in its purity, the public is deeply interested, for it is the foundation of family and society, without which there would be neither civilization nor progress."

Over the course of these past hundred years, the Supreme Court has revisited and reaffirmed this logic. In 1967, for example, in *Loving vs. Virginia*, in striking down a Virginia state law that prohibited interracial marriage, the court reasoned that "marriage is one of the basic civil rights of man, fundamental to our very existence and survival." The citation of cases could be multiplied. For example, the Supreme Court of the United States has refused to elevate various nonmarried relationships to the level of a constitutional right, observing that such conduct is neither "implicit in the concept of ordered liberty" nor "deeply rooted in this nation's history and tradition." In contrast, every state has traditionally encouraged and privileged the marital relationship in recognition of the reality that a stable, lifelong relationship best serves the procreation, care and education of children. This legal tradition is not a matter of private morality and certainly not simply a question of the teaching of the Catholic Church, but rather goes to the very basis of society as a matter of public morality in support of the common good.

It is within this tradition that Harvard Law School Professor Mary Ann Glendon poses the question concerning legislation pertinent to such matters: "What sort of meaning is family law creating and what sort of society is it helping to constitute?"

It is likewise within the framework of Church teaching and the generally consistent traditional religious teaching of other major faith groups, as well as the repetitive court decisions that have verified and been guided by such tradition, that the Church addresses the proposed New York City Domestic Partnership Legislation, Intro. 303. The Church recognizes that it has no right to impose specifically Catholic teaching on others, nor does it desire to do so. The Archdiocese of New York, however, after having had the proposed legislation conscientiously studied by both legal and moral experts, must regrettably conclude that, at least in its current form, the proposed Domestic Partnership Legislation fails to provide the necessary moral and even civil protection for the uniqueness of marriage and family required by its "first and vital cell of society." On the contrary, the proposed legislation may reasonably be interpreted, as, indeed, it has been interpreted, as equating the non-married state with the married state. This cannot, over either the short term or the long term, fail to influence the young in their attitudes toward marriage and family, even discouraging marriage in instances when marriage should be encouraged. It can eventually lead to moral and cultural changes in our society neither anticipated nor traditionally desired from our earliest days as a people.

The Archdiocese of New York comes to this conclusion after examining the proposed legislation, without prejudice to the unmarried. No individual, no class of individuals, merits to be treated unjustly, with contempt or with any other inappropriate response. At the very outset, this statement asserted its assumption of good will on the part of those advocating the proposed legislation, believing that they are currently being deprived of benefits they consider to be their due or that at least these benefits are not currently guaranteed or protected by law. In examining the proposed legislation, then, the Archdiocese makes no judgment on such advocates or their claims. The Archdiocese believes, however, that if human or civil rights are being inappropriately denied, this situation should be addressed in some manner that does not derogate from or appear to derogate from the sanctity and time-honored place of marriage and the family in our society.

The Church believes unconditionally in the uniqueness of the state of marriage defined as the conjugal relationship between a man and a woman, usually recognized in some formal way by the state. The Church believes that such marriage is divinely ordained, so that no human authority can make any other state of life equivalent to marriage. (That this can be said without prejudice toward anyone in any other state of life could be verified by the fact that, even within its own formal religious practices, the Church equates neither a priest nor a religious sister or brother with a married couple. These are simply different states of life.)

Since what has been said here about marriage and family is of dominant concern to the Archdiocese of New York, this statement refrains from addressing other questionable elements of the proposed legislation which legal and moral experts have discerned upon conscientious examination and about which they have advised the Archdiocese. Representatives of the Archdiocese would be prepared to share these findings with those who might be interested and certainly with those who have the responsibility to evaluate the proposed legislation because of their positions. By way of example, however, they have noted that whereas the proposed legislation essentially attempts to establish a parallel form of marriage, it will not be regulated by the domestic relations law, but will have it own set of rules. This could create a number of problems, particularly with regard to how "domestic partners" deal with the state and with third parties. New York state marriages are recognized as valid in other states. What juridical recognition would be given to domestic partners? Would they be recognized in other municipalities? A spouse has a right to support from the other spouse. Will a domestic partner have to provide support? A spouse has certain rights with regard to property. What would be the case in domestic partnerships? What would be the legal effect on children? What of the question of filing joint tax returns, pension rights, etc.? Lawyers examining the proposed legislation have posed these and many other legal questions. Interestingly, they have even asked whether the proposed legislation, intended in part, it appears, to end alleged discrimination against some individuals, does not actually legislate discrimination against others. In sum, the proposed legislation seems burdened with unanswered questions and ambiguities.

Moralists examining the proposed legislation, of course, have understandably raised questions about the morality of extramarital genital relationships, whatever the sex of the parties involved, and have pointed out various other moral issues that they would be prepared to discuss.

In my own judgment, as Archbishop of New York and in accordance with a lifetime of involvement in public policy issues, I have become convinced that the law is one of the most effective teachers in our society. Permit me to quote then-Solicitor General Thurgood Marshall at the White House Conference on Civil Rights in 1966 (Thurgood Marshall, of course, later became a Supreme Court Justice):

> What is striking to me is the importance of law in determining the condition of the Negro. He was effectively enslaved, not by brute force, but by a law which declared him a chattel of his master, who was given the legal right to recapture him even in free territory. He was emancipated by law, and then disenfranchised and segregated by law. And finally he is winning equality by law. . . . Laws not only provide concrete benefit, they can even change the hearts of men, some men anyway, for good or evil.

My conviction about the teaching power and the impact of law even transcends religious teaching. Indeed, I have always been profoundly influenced by the teaching of Cicero, who spoke of law long before the coming of Christ:

> There is in fact a true law, namely right reason, which is in accordance with nature, applies to all men and is unchangeable and eternal. By its commands this law summons men to the performance of their duties, by its prohibitions it restrains them from doing wrong. . . . [T]here will be one law eternal and unchangeable, binding at all times upon all peoples. There will be as it were, one common master and ruler of men, namely God, who is the author of this law, its interpreter and its sponsor. The man who will not obey it will abandon his better self.

It is imperative, in my judgment, that no law be passed contrary to natural moral law and Western tradition by virtually legislating that "marriage does not matter." To refer once again to formal Church teaching, which I, as a Bishop of the Church, am bound to profess and to proclaim, not only religious teachers but also public authorities "should regard it as a sacred duty to recognize, protect, and promote their [marriage and family's] authentic nature, to shield public morality, and to favor the prosperity of domestic life" (*Gaudium et Spes*, 52).

It is precisely because marriage does matter that its authentic nature must be recognized, protected and promoted by society and particularly by government. Marriage matters supremely to every person and every institution in our society. All proposed legislation that might affect the critical status of marriage in our society matters immensely.

We must face the issues of Intro. 303 honestly and try to resolve them justly and charitably. "With malice toward none, with charity toward all," the Archdiocese of New York is open to constructive proposals and is prepared to contribute to honest, just and charitable solutions. May God guide our legislators, members of the City Council, witnesses and all persons of good will in their efforts to come to equitable judgments in regard to the proposed New York City Domestic Partnership Legislation, Intro. 303.

Same-Sex Marriage:
Our Final Answer?

Gerard V. Bradley

In the 1988 edition of his treatise on *The Law of Domestic Relations*, Homer Clark wrote that marriage "is being transformed from a clearly defined relationship" to one whose "incidents are either uncertain or left largely to the control of the parties."[1] Clark's "incidents" included basic elements of marriage (sexual exclusivity, for example),[2] along with secondary attributes and legal effects (such as the property relations of spouses and ex-spouses).[3] Clark opined that the uncertainty and privatization of marriage emerged suddenly, and "without, so far as it appears, any general consideration by either courts or legislatures of the total effect which the judicial decisions will have on the institution of marriage."[4] He wrote a short ten years, by his count, after a time when "it would have been *inconceivable* to deal seriously with the question of the validity of same-sex 'marriage.'"[5] In other words, it was not until 1978 – or later – that the idea of same-sex marriage was even imaginable.

It is surely imaginable now. Vermont recently became the first American jurisdiction to legally recognize same-sex "marriages," calling them (chiefly for political reasons) "civil unions." The Vermont Constitution, as interpreted by the state's highest court in *Baker v. State*,[6] requires an *identity* of legal benefits and protections for *all* couples – opposite- and same-sex – who wish to be married. The court called for legislative action to implement this requirement. The decision held out, however, the possibility that *all* the incidents of marriage could be extended to same-sex couples without calling them *married*. The Vermont legislature, in other words, had to treat them *exactly* as it treated married people. But it could still *say*, if it wished, that it was not recognizing same-sex couples as, legally, "married." The legislators chose this option.[7]

Some observers say that by calling same-sex relationships "civil unions," the legislature forestalled the national day of reckoning which would be thrust upon us by an express same-sex marriage law: whether states which do not recognize same-sex marriages must give "full faith and credit" to marriages from states that do. Put differently, because the U.S. Constitution requires the laws and legal judgments of one state to be given effect in all other states, the question would be: married in Vermont, married everywhere?

The observation – that reckoning is postponed – is mistaken, the product of naivete in some, and of disingenuousness in others. For among the *most* valuable legal benefits and protections of marriage is interstate portability. As Supreme Court Justice Robert Jackson said in the 1948 case, *Estin v. Estin*:

> If there is one thing that the people are entitled to expect from their lawmakers, it is rules of law that will enable individuals to tell whether they are married and, if so, to whom . . . the uncertainties that result are not merely technical; nor are they trivial: the lawfulness of their cohabitation, their children's legitimacy, their title to property, and even whether they are law-abiding persons or criminals.[8]

Jackson wrote, it is true, when it mattered more than it does today with whom one spends the night. But even now the difference between bigamy and lawful marriage can be how well a divorce decree travels. And the many benefits of marriage provide enough incentive for Vermont same-sex couples to seek marital status in states to which they migrate, either temporarily or for the long haul.

Sometime soon a same-sex couple "united" in Vermont will seek to be treated in a destination state – say Indiana, which I call home – as they are treated in Vermont. In that vast majority of jurisdictions which will, for the foreseeable future, maintain *one* legal status for couples – opposite-sex *marriage* – Vermonters will have to be assimilated to it, or, at least allegedly, endure discrimination. Upon discrimination by the first state, our disappointed Vermonters will return to their state's highest court, accurately alleging an *inequality* of benefits and protections: Vermonters Joe and Jill are treated as married elsewhere, but not plaintiffs Joe and Jack. The Vermont legislature will then have no choice but to assimilate same-sex partnerships to the legal status occupied by all other "married" couples in the Green Mountain state. At that point, the Full Faith and Credit question will be inevitable.

All of this may occur before the year is out. It is a near-term certainty. Have we had yet that "general consideration" of the effects upon the "institution of marriage," oddly missing when Clark wrote? What would such a consideration look like? This article examines those two questions.

I
Neutrality

Many people say that they personally believe that marriage is a union of one man and one woman. Many such people are married to persons of the opposite sex, and cannot really imagine the attraction some persons have for others of the same sex. They would be vastly disappointed if one of their children decided that he or she wanted to marry someone of the same sex. They often also say, however, that it would be wrong, perhaps even a grave injustice, for the state to base its law of marriage on a controversial moral judgment, including the judgment – in fact, theirs and that of most people – that marriage is the union of one man and one woman. The thought is that the state ought to be *neutral* as between competing understandings of what marriage is. It would be wrong, these persons say, for the state to impose *anyone's* moral code for marriage, to make my, or your, morality the template impressed upon all.

Sometimes this viewpoint is elaborated along the following lines. Marriage is, in truth, the union of a man and a woman, as Scripture teaches. Marriage is a sacrament (or an analogous sacred relationship) in many religions. But, although it is the truth about marriage, the religious provenance of this definition makes it an inappropriate basis for civil law. Along these lines, one could say that marriage really is permanent; divorce is impermissible or even, strictly speaking, impossible. But one could coherently say as well that civil law ought not to track this view by making no provision for divorce.

About this way of viewing the relationship of the truth about marriage and the civil law, I make the following three preliminary points. First, on no one's account of it (as far as I know) is the civil law supposed to simply reproduce the moral truth about marriage. Much of what is truly good in and about marriage is beyond effective legal assistance. The endless self-giving that is required of spouses could scarcely be legally enforced. Everyone is a bad spouse sometimes, and some persons are bad spouses most of the time. Still, no one suggests that there should be legal penalties for being a bad (ungenerous, self-centered, indifferent) spouse. Men who see more of professional football than they do their wives and children combined will have a lot to answer for on Judgment Day – in the hereafter, not here.

The most that anyone proposes is that the civil law ought to reflect some basic or defining features of marriage, and only where that serves political society's common good.[9] To what extent the law ought to make provision for civil divorce is, it seems to me, a question permitting a range of answers consistent with the moral truth that a valid marriage is indissoluble. A legal regime of "no-fault divorce," though, seems outside that range. But one need not take a strong view of the permanence of marriage to hold that no-fault divorce has worked great harm to innocent people in our society, and that some type of fault regime would be a great benefit.

Second, the common mindset described above suffers from what I call the "transparency" problem. When speaking of one's judgment that, for example, same-sex marriage is wrong or impossible, one is often heard to say that it is "my" view, or part of "my" moral code," or that it is something one can't help believing, a matter of feeling or irrational commitment. This way of speaking is often an innocent way of saying that same-sex marriage is simply wrong, objectively. This way of speaking is harmful, however, when casually (often unthinkingly) joined to ambient notions of moral subjectivism or emotivitism. Then, when one says that coercion based upon "my" morality would be an unfair imposition, one is *right*. For the *fact* that a judgment is *mine* – one I can't help believing – is not a *reason* for the state to act in a certain way, perhaps especially to the detriment of others who do not share *my* view. That one feels repulsed by what homosexuals do is not a reason for public policy. It is not a reason at all. It is just a feeling.

But no one really thinks that the fact of holding a view is a reason for action, apart from the *reasons* why one holds the view to be true. Thus, in contrast to the opaque or intransitive quality of moral judgment evident in the common view expressed above, conclusions about the morality of same-sex marriage usually are, and should generally be seen as, *transparent* for the reasons *why* the view is held. Some people may be able to give no account of their reasons, and they will make uninteresting conversation parties. Some people really are moral emotivists or relativists, and *would* be unfairly imposing upon others if they caused the state to act coercively on the basis of their feelings. But these facts about some people do not support the proposition that opposition to same-sex marriage is necessarily, or even commonly, subjective, or emotive.

Most people believe and mean to say that same-sex marriage is simply wrong for everyone, that it is objectively and categorically immoral. This view could be false. If it is, its falsity is sufficient reason to discard it. Then doctrines about political "neutrality" or unjust imposition are unnecessary. If the view is true, then such doctrines are either inapposite, or require argument in their favor.

Third, the common mindset asserts or implies that certain truths about marriage (such as its permanence or heterosexuality) can be known *only* due to revelation or because of the authority of a sacred text or religious personality. The view asserts or implies that they are *not* knowable by reason alone. Some defenses of legal recognition of same-sex marriage, notably the Hawaii Supreme Court decision examined below, appear to take this view. If this account is true, I agree that the civil law should be not founded upon such esoteric truths. But the Hawaii court baldly *asserted* the non-rational, and (evidently) the sectarian, province of the heterosexuality of marriage. Assertions will not do; nor will simple dismissals.

Now, note well: the claim that the law *ought* to be morally neutral about marriage, or anything else for that matter, is itself a moral claim. It – the claim that the law *ought* to be neutral – is not morally neutral. As Princeton Professor Robert George points out, anyone who holds that the civil provisions governing marriage (or any other institution or practice) ought to be morally neutral does not assert, nor does the position presuppose, that the law ought to be neutral as between the view that the law ought to be neutral and competing moral views.[10] It is "obvious," he says, "that neutrality between neutrality and non-neutrality is logically impossible."[11]

Besides, even a practical neutrality is impossible. There is good reason to hold that the meaning and significance of marriage are available, in any effective and widespread way emphasis on: only where the host culture, including its law, embodies and encourages a sound understanding of marriage. As Professor George states:

> [Where] ideologies and practices which are hostile to a sound understanding and practice of marriage in a culture tend to undermine the institution of marriage in that culture, thus making it difficult for large numbers of people to grasp the true meaning, value, and significance of marriage, it is extremely important that government eschew attempts to be "neutral" with regard to competing conceptions of marriage and try hard to embody in its law and policy the soundest, most nearly correct conception.[12]

The civil law, even in societies like ours in which people often profess "neutrality," is still a potent teacher. The law will inevitably teach *some* lesson about what marriage is, and what parties to marriage can or should expect from it. It may *seem* that the law is innocent of such aspirations, and bereft of such presuppositions. It may *seem* that marriage, viewed legally, is all form without substance. It may *seem* that the law teaches only the lesson articulated by Homer Clark: marriage is tailor-made to suit the parties to it, and that the function and purpose of marriage law is to facilitate the choices of the individuals who are getting married. It may *seem* that Justice Brennan captured our notions in the *Michael H.* case:

> Even if we can agree, therefore, that "family" and "parenthood" are part of the good life, it is absurd to assume that we can agree on the content of those terms and destructive to pretend that we do. In a community such as ours, "liberty" must include the freedom not to conform.[13]

All these expressions suggest that the state can, and should, recognize and endorse marriage – if only by bestowing some three hundred or so incidental benefits – without *any* specific definition of the relationship, and evidently without using evaluative criteria.

It is impossible to imagine an institution, however, with as many legal benefits as marriage, having (or proponents of the institution and its concomitant benefits, having) no self-understanding, no parameters, no extra-legal presuppositions or commitments. It would be bizarre, and very likely unjust, to impose the costs of such benefits and protections upon society's members without an answer to the question, Why? How is the cost justified? What is marriage, and why is it so special? No answer is possible without *some* definition of marriage, and without *some* theory of *that* relationship to its parties, and to political society.

We find, unsurprisingly then, that legal stories about marriage always contain *some* statement about why marriage is valuable. Homer Clark said: "the fact is that the most significant function of marriage today seems to be that it furnishes emotional satisfactions to be found in no other relationships. For many people it is a refuge from the coldness and impersonality of contemporary existence."[14] Maybe so. But upon what basis is *this* particular part of marriage picked out from among all its parts, held up as especially salient to deliberation by public authority, and deemed sufficient to justify the regime of special treatment we accord marriage? Mark Strasser, in *Legally Wed: Same-sex Marriage and the Constitution*, argues that the state has "a responsibility to recognize" the "intensely personal bonds" between committed homosexuals.[15] Again, why should "intensely personal bonds" be the *sine qua non* of marriage, and upon what basis does the state have a "responsibility" to endorse them? Why not the "intensely personal bonds" between siblings? Of close, but not sexually involved, friends?

Joseph Raz, who does not take the negative view of same-sex marriage that I do, nevertheless correctly states the relation between the law of marriage and the real-world possibilities for participation in the good of marriage: "[M]onogamy, assuming that it is the only valuable form of marriage, cannot be practiced by an individual. It requires a culture which recognizes it, and which supports it through the public's attitude and through its formal institutions."[16]

Raz does not suppose that, in a culture whose law and public morality do not support monogamy, someone who happens to believe in it somehow will be unable to restrict himself to having one wife or will be required to take additional wives.[17] His point, rather, is

> [E]ven if monogamy is a key element of a sound understanding of marriage, large numbers of people will fail to understand that or why that is the case – and will therefore fail to grasp the value of monogamy and the intelligible point of practicing it – unless they are assisted by a culture which supports monogamous marriage. Marriage is the type of good which can be participated in, or fully participated in, only by people who properly understand it and choose it with a proper understanding in mind; yet people's ability properly to understand it, and thus to

choose it, depends upon institutions and cultural understandings that transcend individual choice.[18]

II
Equality

Some arguments for legal recognition of same-sex marriage, though phrased in terms of equality, actually depend upon the validity of (presupposed) neutrality claims. Stephen Macedo, who supports same-sex marriage, says that the law of marriage denies "fundamental aspects of equality" by embodying the moral judgment that marriage is inherently heterosexual.[19] But this is sound only if it is false that marriage is inherently heterosexual. If that view is false, the reason for recognizing same-sex marriages is that such unions are, as a matter of moral fact, indistinguishable from marriages of the traditional type. If the moral judgment is true, then Macedo's claim that the recognition of this truth by government "denies fundamental aspects of equality" is simply mistaken.[20]

In *Bowers v. Hardwick*,[21] (a 1986 case about whether homosexuals have a Constitutional right to commit sodomy), Justice Harry Blackmun suggested an intriguing argument, based in equality, for legal recognition of same-sex marriage. The context in *Bowers*, of course, was not same-sex marriage but homosexual sexual acts. Blackmun's notion of equal respect for the foundation of a person's identity and essential acts in conformity therewith nevertheless seems – if sound – potent enough to carry the case for recognition of same-sex marriage.

The Court resolved in *Bowers* that Georgia could, consistent with the Constitution, make the sodomitical acts of homosexuals a crime. In the course of his dissent from that holding, Justice Blackmun referred to "homosexual orientation" as "the very fiber of an individual's personality," a fiber not "simply a matter of deliberate personal election."[22] In other words, at least some homosexuals find themselves inescapably attracted to persons of the same sex. This attraction, Blackmun implied, constitutes a – if not *the* – foundation of such persons' identities. And, if marriage is considered the setting in which sexual acts are appropriate, then (as Blackmun said in *Bowers*) the homosexual "is given no real choice but a life without physical intimacy."[23] *This*, Blackmun left to inevitable inference, was both cruel and unequal, more than anyone should be asked to bear, more than heterosexuals are asked to bear.

Blackmun seems to be assuming that everyone is entitled to regular (albeit "harmless") satisfaction of the sexual urge. On all these assumptions, then, there *is* a denial of some sort of "equality" where, at least as far as formal legal treatment is concerned, the state recognizes no legitimate sexual outlet for homosexuals.

The answer is this. Persons do constitute their identities. But they do not do so by identifying some sub-rational drive (like "sexual orientation"), but through free choices. Some homosexuals may not choose to be homosexual. But they can and do choose to be "gay" or "lesbian"; that is, they choose to identify themselves as not only persons with a same-sex attraction but as "gay": homosexual *and* approving of same-sex sexual activity.

Blackmun's argument fails for another reason, too. To expect others to "respect" or in any way endorse someone as "gay" is to *require* them to give sodomy a positive moral value. *This* expectation, often expressed as a demand, indicates a lack of respect for all others who regard sodomy as immoral. Thus "homophobia" is treated as racism deserves to be treated.

In truth nothing in opposition to legal recognition of same-sex marriage intends or implies insult to homosexuals or a denial of equality of respect and concern toward them. The equality of all persons is an equality of dignity, which means that each one's good is as good as everyone else's. And one shows respect and concern for homosexuals precisely by declining to accord sodomy a moral value it simply does not possess.

III
Arbitrariness

Another type of equality argument has much appeal, and it is time to examine it. It is not so much about law as about culture, or about the condition of marriage in our society. The examination is especially important because the structure of this argument, though not all its content, persuaded the high courts of Vermont and Hawaii to (effectively) recognize same-sex marriage.

The argument, in outline form, is this. What most heterosexual couples seek and obtain from marriage – and thus what they consider marriage to be – depends in no significant way upon their heterosexuality; same-sex couples can and do obtain the same things from their committed relationships. Many same-sex couples consider their relationships to be marital, and desire legal recognition of their relationships as marriage. This desire includes but is not limited to the attraction and utility of tangible benefits legally available to married couples. Like most opposite-sex couples, same-sex couples find the state's recognition an endorsement of sorts, a welcome perfection of, or intangible supplement to, their unions. The conclusion: it is *arbitrary* to deny recognition to same-sex relationships. Lacking as it does a reasonable basis, denial of recognition probably rests upon some irrational prejudice toward homosexuals. Either way – as arbitrary or as hateful – exclusion of same-sex couples from the legal regime inhabited by opposite-sex couples is unconstitutional.

There is *much* to be said in favor of this argument. After all, this far down the road of "transformation" charted by Homer Clark, what *do* many (most?) men and women assent to when they say "I do." Many (most?) mean to set up and manage a household, more or less throwing their financial lots together. They agree to try hard at an emotionally intimate, sexually active relationship, hopefully lasting and, ideally, sexually exclusive. Children? Maybe, eventually. But for now, sodomitical acts and acts of contracepted intercourse make for a mutually agreeable, pleasurable sex life.

Homer Clark is once again a reliable witness.

> It seems to be that contemporary marriage cannot be legally defined any more precisely than as some sort of relationship between two individuals, of indeterminate duration, involving some kind of sexual conduct, entailing vague mutual property and support obligations, a relationship which may be formed by

Gerard V. Bradley

consent of both parties and dissolved at the will of either.[24]

On this common view, men and women entering marriage intend principally personal benefits to themselves: sexual satisfaction, emotional intimacy and support, mutual sharing of household duties, and (perhaps) children. But same-sex couples can and do obtain these same benefits. They can even have children, though not of their own union. They can adopt, sometimes the natural children of one partner from a marriage which went bad after the partner discovered his or her homosexuality. Or, if the couple is male, they can contract with a woman friend or acquaintance or stranger to bear the child of one of them. If the couple is female, one can impregnate herself, either through the services of a sperm bank or of a more intimate donor.

This argument is that it is not coherent with marriage as it is really *practiced* by Americans for the people – and their representatives exercising public authority – to say that committed homosexual relationships are not, and cannot be, marriages. One obvious counter-argument is that opposite-sex couples can express or actualize something in their sexual acts which same-sex couples cannot: marriage. Since same-sex couples cannot marry they cannot be doing the same thing that married couples do, insofar as married couples experience in their marital acts, in addition to pleasure and emotional benefits, the intelligible good of their marriage itself. It simply is the case, the counter-argument holds, that same-sex couples *cannot*, and *never* will be able to, engage in the reproductive type acts – sexual intercourse, open to the gift of new life – that married couples can perform.

This counter-argument is question-begging. *Why* cannot same-sex couples marry, where marriage is not, as it seems not to be in our legal culture, tied to openness to children? After all, sterile couples are permitted to marry, and many fertile couples with no present interest in having children get married, too.

A full response to this challenge requires careful elaboration of precisely how marriage is a reproductive communion of persons, a two-in-one-flesh lifetime friendship which, as such, is available only to persons of the opposite sex. That elaboration is to be found in Part VI of this Chapter. In advance of that full discussion, however, we can see that this argument from coherence is not as persuasive as it first appears.

There is nothing unbecoming in arguments, like the one just sketched, which identify an apparent arbitrariness in "straight" monopolization of marriage. But the picture just presented is only part of the story. Additional pertinent facts include that, at least for male homosexuals, "committed" relationships are very rarely lasting, and almost never sexually exclusive. There is abundant evidence that neither permanence nor sexual exclusivity are considered norms even by those (perhaps relatively few) male homosexuals who are in committed relationships. There appears to be very little support, at least among male homosexuals, for *monogamy* even as a norm, as heterosexuals and our law understand it: complete sexual fidelity; no outside sexual satisfaction whatsoever.

It is true, as the incoherence argument for same-sex marriage alleges, that many married couples today are ambivalent about having children. Many married couples today do, in fact, engage in completed sexual acts other than intercourse. But even these couples recognize the difference, not just in the physical performance, but in the way in which their marriage is experienced, between sodomy and sexual intercourse, especially where the couple do nothing to impede whatever procreative possibilities inhere in that act of intercourse. Simply put, marital acts in which the couple places hopes of having a baby are experienced by that couple as different, especially fulfilling acts, just from the point of view of allowing them to experience their marriage.

Sterility is not considered a blessing upon a couple's marriage. To a greater or lesser degree it is experienced by the vast majority of sterile couples as a loss, as a deprivation. Children do not "complete" a marriage in the sense that a marriage is not official or valid until children are born. (Otherwise, every one of us who is a firstborn would have been conceived out of wedlock.) Childless couples are really married. But compared to a sterile couple who have adopted children, the couple which conceives and brings forth children from its own marital acts perfects their marriage in an unsurpassable way.

The *massive* discordant fact simply is this: most Americans do not believe that people can marry a person of the same sex. That means that most Americans hold that gender complementarity is, somehow, essential to marriage. If that does not indicate a popular conviction at odds with the arbitrariness argument, I cannot imagine what would.

We can see, then, that the practical predicate to the incoherence argument is faulty. There is also a logical flaw in the argument; people do not accept all that is entailed by their premises. Few are aware of all that their premises lead to, and many do not know much of what is entailed. Now is their opportunity to see what premises are necessary to defend what they still hold to be true – that marriage is the more or less permanent and exclusive union of one man and one woman, and that this relationship is the principle of all sexual morality. Once the two coherent accounts of sexual morality are fully sketched – and only then – can the American people actually *decide* whether they wish to conform their practices to the true nature of marriage, or to release the law's understanding of marriage from its foundation in gender complementarity.

IV
Courts

The argument from popular or cultural arbitrariness is overdrawn. A structurally similar argument nevertheless persuaded the Vermont Supreme Court that discrimination against same-sex couples was inconsistent with that state constitution's "common benefits" clause. The argument advanced by the court aimed to show that Vermont maintains no *coherent* legal view of marriage which could justify excluding same-sex couples from its benefits. The rejoinder is also similar to that proposed against the cultural argument from inequality: the law of marriage may, up to a significant point, be incoherent. But this fact of incoherence makes the *question* of what the law of marriage should be all the more acute. It does not *settle*, by force of logic, what the law is. We can see in the Vermont court's opinion the effects of Clark's observations: the law of marriage stands at a dangerously high precipice, pushed there by proponents of same-sex. *Now* is the time for that consideration, already overdue when Clark wrote in 1988.

The Vermont court held that all legal benefits must be uniformly distributed, save where the exclusion of some persons "bears a reasonable and just relation to the governmental purpose" of the benefit program.[25] The Court observed that "the benefits and protections incident to a marriage license under Vermont law have never been greater,"[26] and that "any statutory exclusion must necessarily be grounded on public concerns of sufficient weight, cogency, and authority that the justice of the deprivation cannot seriously be questioned."[27] Notice the starting point: equality dictates that everyone, at least presumptively, is eligible to receive the benefits of marriage. It looks, then, like the benefits are *prima facie* constitutive of the class of beneficiaries: anyone who would be (or thinks he would be) better off with the benefits is presumptively entitled to get married, so as to recive the benefits!

The State was on the right track in its justification for limiting marital benefits to opposite sex couples. Its interest was the link between marriage, procreation, and child rearing. In probably the Court's most sympathetic statement of this interest, the stated aim was to promote a "permanent commitment between couples who have children to ensure that their offspring are considered legitimate," receive "ongoing parental support,"[28] and that there be a sustained public message that child rearing is "intertwined" with the procreative acts of man and woman married to each other.

The Court responded along the lines of the arbitrariness argument. "It is equally undisputed that many *opposite*-sex couples marry for reasons unrelated to procreation, that some of these couples never intend to have children, and that others are incapable of having children."[29] If the purpose of the statutory exclusion of same-sex couples is to "further the link between procreation and child rearing,"the Court concluded, it is significantly under-inclusive.[30] The law extends the benefits and protections of marriage to many persons with no logical connection to the stated governmental goal.[31] Therefore, "the statutes plainly exclude many same-sex couples who are no different from opposite-sex couples with respect to these objectives."[32]

The State also argued that "because same-sex couples cannot conceive a child on their own, their exclusion promotes a "perception of the link between procreation and child rearing," The court responded: "Indeed, it is undisputed that most of those who utilize nontraditional means of conception are infertile *married* couples."[33] Hence the law's acceptance of certain reproductive technologies making conception independent of marital intercourse undermined the case against same-sex marriage. But as the last quoted sentence suggests, the non-prohibition of such acts as artificial insemination probably owes much to a desire by those responsible for the law to *extend* the reproductive meaning of marriage to couples unable to generate children from their own acts of intercourse, not, as the court seems to have concluded, to obliterate the (central) reproductive meaning of marriage.

The State's remaining claims were undone by another concession, this time to same-sex couples themselves. "The Legislature could conclude," wrote the Court, "that opposite-sex partners offer advantages" in the area of "childrearing." After noting "that child-development experts disagree and the answer is decidedly uncertain," the Court moved on to the "fundamental flaw": the "legislature's endorsement of a policy diametrically at odds with the State's claim." That policy was the removal, in 1996, of all legal barriers to the adoption of children by same-sex couples.[34]

But: that same-sex couples may adopt implies only that the particular two people are acceptable parents. It does not imply that they can marry. Many single persons adopt children, and that implies nothing about marriage. That same-sex couples may adopt, moreover, implies *nothing* positive or favorable about their sexual identity and activities. Two persons of the same sex, though not a sexually involved couple, could probably serve as adoptive parents, too. This is very likely the description under which "same-sex couples" are permitted to adopt, in Vermont and elsewhere. It is doubtful that Vermont accepted adoption by sexually involved same-sex couples *because* of their sexual relationship. One simply cannot deduce from the fact that same-sex couples may adopt that, *as gay*, they are thought to be fit parents, or that one can marry his or her same-sex partner.

Finally, but most important, *if* accepting adoption by same-sex couples *entailed* same-sex marriage, those who accepted same-sex-couples adoption very likely did not think so. *Now* they should be given the opportunity to decide whether, if *that* is what is entailed, they wish to retract the permission to adopt. Instead the Vermont Supreme Court made sure that the issue of same-sex marriage was never really decided: The Court basically said that there is no alternative *now* – because of decisions *then* – to recognition of same-sex marriage. But there is no evidence, and certainly none was adduced by the Vermont court, that *then* anyone was then expressing any view, much less a favorable one, about same-sex marriage.

A continent away, and a few years before *Baker v. State*, the Hawaii Supreme Court engaged in another evasive validation of same-sex marriage. What did the Hawaii Supreme Court, in the case of Ninia Baehr (who wanted to marry Genora Dancel) versus John Lewin (the state official responsible for denying Baehr a marriage license), say?[35] Probably not what you think it did. One would expect from all that was reported about this decision that Hawaiian same-sex marriage is "gay marriage," with its implicit approval of homosexual sexual activity. Hawaiian same-sex marriage turns out to be no-sex marriage. The Hawaii Supreme Court (strongly) observed: "'Homosexual' and 'same-sex' marriages are not synonymous; by the same token, a 'heterosexual' same-sex marriage is, in theory, not oxymoronic. . . . Parties to 'a union between a man and a woman' may or may not be homosexuals. Parties to a same-sex marriage could be either homosexuals or heterosexuals."[36] The court later said that "it is immaterial" whether "the plaintiffs [that is, the same-sex couples, including Baehr and Doncel] are homosexuals."[37] The court also pointed out that nowhere did the plaintiffs say they were homosexual (or, heterosexual, for that matter).[38]

The Hawaii Supreme Court discussed at length what most people have in mind when they speak of marriage. But this marriage the court associated with the right of privacy located somewhere in the federal constitution, and called it the "federal construct" of marriage. It, the court correctly reported, "presently contemplates unions between men and women," and is associated with or defined by the "fundamental rights of procreation, child-birth, abortion, and child rearing."[39] (Yes, the court *did* say that "abortion" is part of the definition of marriage, a proposition which would surprise most people. And what the court meant by its assertion of this heterogeneous bundle and the "federal" right to marry as "the logical predicate[s]" of each other is anyone's guess.)

We can see that Hawaiian marriage swings free of the "federal construct," and of the idea that one essential feature of marriage is that it is a sexual, indeed reproductive, union. Let's call this, simply, marriage. Hawaiian "marriage" is radically divorced from it. The estrangement is most vividly illustrated in the court's response to arguments advanced on behalf of Lewin. The state, as the court related the point, "contends that 'the fact that homosexual [*sic* – actually, same-sex] partners cannot form a state-licensed marriage is not the product of impermissible discrimination' implicating equal protection considerations, but rather 'a function of their biologic inability as a couple to satisfy the definition of the status to which they aspire.'"[40] The argument is, in other words, that given what marriage really – metaphysically, morally, pre-legally – is, persons of the same gender simply cannot marry. "We believe," said the court, that the argument is "circular and unper-suasive," "an exercise in tortured and conclusory sophistry."[41]

The court's "belie[f]" amounted to a simple declaration that it would not hear, in a case raising the legal recognition of same-sex marriages, arguments about what marriage *is*. And so the Hawaii Supreme Court articulated and imposed upon the people of that state an unsurpassably positivistic definition of marriage, one which could be related to the moral reality of the matter by, evidently, only a sadistic sophist. The court's "marriage" was, in principle, sexless, and almost all about money. Calling it revealingly at one point a "legal partnership," the court listed fourteen specific benefits to which this "legally conferred status" is the gatekeeper. Twelve of them were clearly economic advantages; the other two – easier name changing and the evidentiary privilege for spousal communication – were relatively minor.

V
Getting the Question Right

The Hawaii court got the fundamental question backwards. One should not imagine – as the court did – that the law attaches certain benefits to the status of "marriage" without *first* determining *that* there is a specific relationship which *deserves* such beneficial treatment. One should not imagine that lawmakers ever decided to create an entitlement program with various goodies to be distributed, and then decided to call it (for some reason) "marriage," with the idea of making eligibility (to be "married") functionally related to the benefits. *If* you can enjoy the benefits, you can get married. On this view, "marriage" is an empty placeholder in a social welfare scheme.

There is no room to doubt that the legal regime – of benefits, protections and duties – which has surrounded marriage since our founding got its start from the opposite direction. Marriage has regularly been said to be subject to legal regulation. But the central thrust of the many political, especially judicial, testimonies to the value of marriage has been the salutary effects this pre-political (and thus natural) institution has upon the fortunes of political society, and upon the happiness of people. For these reasons marriage has been thought worthy of extensive social and legal support.

Two examples of the long traditional judicial testimony will have to suffice. In *Maynard v. Hill*[42] the U.S. Supreme Court said that marriage creates "the most important relation in life" and has "more to do with the morals and civilization of a people than any other institution."[43] Marriage also, the Court said, "is the foundation of the family and of society, without which there would be neither civilization or progress."[44]

Why? In 1961, Justice Harlan explained, though in a summary way, *why* marriage – the union of one man and one woman – occupies this central place:

> [T]he very inclusion of the category of morality among state concerns indicates that society is not limited in its objects only to the physical well-being of the

> community, but has traditionally concerned itself with the moral soundness of its people as well. . . . The laws regarding marriage which provide both when the sexual powers may be used and the legal and societal context in which children are born and brought up, as well as laws forbidding adultery, fornication and homosexual practices which express the negative of the proposition, confining sexuality to lawful marriage, a pattern deeply pressed into the substance of our social life form[s].[45]

Here are the two features of marriage which lawmakers from time out of mind have picked out of that complex open-ended relationship as *critically* important to the political common good: marriage as the principle of sexual morality, and marriage as the only legitimate setting in which children should come to be, and be raised. It has surely been the undoing of marriage that, as a society, we have detached both sex and marriage from children.

VI
Getting the Answer Right

Contemporary common sense, as well as our legal and moral traditions, point us to the existence of some decisive relation among marriage, children and how children come to be.[46] The practical insight that marriage has its own intelligible point, and that it is a one-flesh communion of persons consummated and actualized in the reproductive-type acts of spouses, cannot be attained by someone who has no idea of what these terms mean; nor can it be attained, except with strenuous efforts of imagination, by people who, due to personal or cultural circumstances, have little acquaintance with actual marriages thus understood. For this reason, whatever undermines the sound understanding and practice of marriage in a culture – including ideologies that are hostile to that understanding and practice – makes it difficult for people to grasp the intrinsic value of marriage and marital intercourse.

Although much in our culture has tended in recent years to undermine the institution of marriage and the moral understandings upon which it rests, longstanding features of our legal and religious traditions testify to the intrinsic value of marriage as a two-in-one-flesh communion. Consummation has traditionally (though, perhaps, not universally) been recognized by civil as well as religious authorities as an essential element of marriage. Pre-existing, incurable physical defects and incapacities which render a party unable to consummate the marriage, are, under most statutes, grounds for annulment. This requirement for the validity of a marriage, where in force, has never been treated as satisfied by an act of sodomy, no matter how pleasurable. Nothing less (or more) than an act of genital union consummates a marriage; and such an act consummates even if it is not particularly pleasurable. Unless otherwise impeded, couples who know they are sterile can lawfully marry so long as they are capable of consummating their marriage by performing such an act. By the same token, a marriage cannot be annulled for want of consummation on the ground that one of the spouses turned out to be sterile. A marriage can, however, be annulled on the ground that impotence (or some other condition) prevents the partners from consummating it.

The law, in its rules regarding consummation, embodies an important insight into the nature of marriage as a bodily – no less than spiritual and emotional – union that is actualized in reproductive-type acts. Some people, however, may well consider the law simply to be misguided on this point. Marriage, they may argue, is a one-flesh union only in a metaphorical sense. It is, in reality, they may say, an emotional union that is served in various ways by the mutually satisfying orgasmic acts of spouses. Consummation, they may contend, ought not to be a requirement for the validity of marriage, or, if it is to be a requirement, it should be considered to have been satisfied by a wider range of possible sexual behaviors.

In the end, one either understands that spousal genital intercourse has a special significance as instantiating a basic, non-instrumental value, or something blocks that understanding and one does not perceive correctly. For the most part, proponents of same-sex marriage honestly do not see any special point or value in such intercourse. For them, spouses have no reason, apart from

Gerard V. Bradley

purely subjective preference, ever to choose genital intercourse over oral and anal intercourse. And because oral and anal intercourse are available to same-sex couples, such couples have as much interest in marriage and as much right to marry as couples of opposite sexes.

By contrast, many other people perceive quite easily the special value and significance of the genital intercourse of spouses, and see that this value and significance obtains even for spouses who are incapable of having children, or any more children. They are therefore confident that sodomitical acts cannot be marital (though they divide over the question whether contracepted intercourse retains its marital quality). Thus, as a matter of common sense, they deny that marriage, as a moral reality, is possible for couples of the same sex.

In my view, children conceived in marital intercourse participate in the good of their parents' marriage and are themselves noninstrumental aspects of its perfection; thus, spouses rightly hope for and welcome children, not as "products" they "make," but rather, as gifts, which if all goes well, supervene on their acts on marital union. This understanding of children as gifts to be accepted and valued for their own sake – rather than as objects that may be willed and brought into being for one's own purposes – obviously coheres well with certain theistic metaphysical views, including Jewish and Christian views. It can, however, also be accommodated by Buddhist and certain other nontheistic views. Some understanding along these lines of the moral relationship of parents to the children they may conceive is essential to the rational affirmation of the dignity of children as *persons:* i.e., as *ends in themselves*, and not mere *means* of satisfying desires of their parents; as *subjects* of justice (including fundamental and inviolable human rights), rather than objects of will. Alternative understandings run into severe difficulties in explaining why children may not properly be understood – and rightly treated – as the property of their parents.

Some people are puzzled by the tendency of moral traditionalists to object on moral grounds to the production of human beings by *in vitro* fertilization. After all, the moral tradition strongly affirms the goodness of transmitting life to new persons. Why, then, should couples who are incapable of begetting children in acts of marital intercourse not resort to *in vitro* processes in order to become parents? The short answer is that the manufacturing of children is inconsistent with respect for their basic equality and human dignity.

Children are to be desired under a description that does not reduce the child to the status of a product to be brought into existence at its parents' will and for their ends. Children rather are to be treated as *persons* – possessing full human dignity – which the spouses are eager to welcome (and take responsibility for) as a perfective participant in the community established by their marriage (i.e., their family). (It is in this sense that one speaks of children as "gifts" that "supervene" on marital acts.) This is not to suggest that there is anything wrong with spouses engaging in marital intercourse because they "want" a child. It is merely to indicate the description under which the "wanting" of the child is consistent with his or her dignity as a person, and to highlight the fact that the marital significance of properly motivated spousal intercourse obtains whether or not conception is hoped for, results, or is even possible. Importantly, however, the intrinsic worth and dignity of a child is in no way diminished by any moral defect in the act that brings that child into existence

VII
Homosexuality and the Common Good

Some critics of the view I have defended here assert that it relegates, at least by implication, homosexuals to second-class citizenship. This criticism is wide of the mark. The truth is that homosexuality is irrelevant to almost every question pertaining to the common good of political society. That is partly because the most important civil rights are human rights. Human rights attach to everyone because they are human persons. These rights do not acquire their sense, and vary not at all in their precise content, according upon one's "sexual orientation," or, for that matter, on the state of one's character in regard to other matters, such as justice.

Homosexuality is almost entirely irrelevant partly because people are to be morally judged on the basis of their conduct, not their condition. Simply being homosexual is not, and should not be, the basis of criminal liability because being homosexual is not an act. Similarly, it is wrong to think of "punishing" (a moral category) anyone for being homosexual, or for any other unjust attitude or desire.

Finally, homosexuality is almost entirely irrelevant to how persons should be treated by civil authority because most of the particular rights and duties of political and civil life do not implicate one's sexual activity, habits or orientation – whatever they may be. Eligibility for driver's licenses, for library privileges, to sit as jurors; duties to pay taxes, observe the speed limit, and to avoid harms to others have their sources in skills, opportunities and moral norms which do not include sexual inclination or activity in any way, for anyone. "Heterosexuals" (as such) are no more, and no less eligible, for jury service than "homosexuals" (as such) are.

The law does not condemn homosexuals to loneliness, nor does it discriminate against same-sex friendships. The law has always regarded genuine friendship, apart from family ties and sexual intimacy, as good grounds for some legal relations. Any two people can sign a lease or take out a loan together. Anyone may be given power of attorney, be appointed guardian ad litem, executor of an estate. The law presumes that trusted others – friends – will fill such important legal slots. Friendship therefore has a vital place in the good life, a place recognized and facilitated by our law.

Marriage, it is true, is a type of friendship. The argument of Part VI is that marriage is a *unique* type of friendship, specified by the capacity to engage in reproductive type acts, which is simply unavailable to same-sex couples.

Conclusion

Have we had that "general consideration" of marriage which Homer Clark called for in 1988? No. The "transformation" he describes now has reached a climactic stage. We are in the twilight of the monumental struggle over marriage, and therefore, about sexual morality and the terms and conditions under which children come to be. The conclusive separation of marriage from its millennia-old identification with reproductive-type acts – and thus with gender complementarity – is the question acutely posed by same-sex marriage. Yet the argument has not really been joined. The arguments for this revolutionary change either beg the question, or treat the conclusion as settled by deduction, or strong inference, from established premises. It is true that discordant elements have been introduced, as Clark testified, into marriage but (as he further says) without really thinking about it. Now that incoherence is said to preclude deliberation and debate on the matter further. The question was settled, in other words, without anyone actually asking – much less answering – it. On a matter so fundamental as this, that should not be our final answer.

Endnotes

1. H. Clark, The Law of Domestic Relations in the United States, 31 (2nd ed.1988).

2. See id at 27.

3. See id at 29.

4. Id. at 31.

5. Id. at 75. Emphasis added.

6. 744 A. 2d 864 (1999).

7. 1999 Vt. Acts and Resolves 847 (enacted April 26, 2000).

8. Estin v. Estin, 334 U.S. 541 (1948) (Jackson, J. dissenting).

9. It is important to note here that "common good" should not be understood along the utilitarian lines. The common good of political society includes a decent concern for public morality and, as we shall see, maintenance of conditions which help people to understand what marriage is and to succeed in the marriages they enter into.

10. See R. George, "'Same-sex Marriage' and 'Moral Neutrality'" (unpublished paper on file with author). Much of the next few paragraphs follows Professor George's argument.

11. Id. at 23.

12. R. George, supra note 11, at 23.

13. Michael H. v. Gerald D., 491 U.S. 110, 141 (1989).

Gerard V. Bradley

14. Clark, supra note 1, at 28.
15. Mark Strasser, Legally Wed: Same-sex Marriage and the Constitution.
16. Joseph Raz, The Morality of Freedom (Oxford: Clarendon Press, 1986), p. 162.
17. See George, supra note 11, at 24.
18. Raz, supra note 21, at 162.
19. Macedo, supra note 14, at 335.
20. See George, supra note 11, at 23.
21. 478 U.S. 186 (1986).
22. Id. at 202–3 n.2 (Blackmun J, dissenting).
23. Id.
24. Clark, supra note 1, at 28.
25. Baker v. State, 744 A 2d 864, 879 (1999).
26. Id at 883.
27. Id at 884.
28. Id. at 881.
29. Id.
30. Id.
31. See id. at 88.
32. Id. at 882.
33. Id.
34. Id. at 884 (for all quotations in paragraph).
34. See Baehr v. Lewin, 852 P. 2d 44 (1993).
36. Id. 51 n. 11.
37. Id. at 53 n. 14.
38. See id.
39. Id at 60.
40. Id.
41. Id. at 61.
42. 125 U.S. 190 (1888).
43. Id. at 211.
44. Id.

45. Poe v. Ullman, 367 U.S. 497, 545-46 (1961) (Harlan J., dissenting).

46. Much of this part is based upon Robert P. George and Gerard V. Bradley, "Marriage and the Liberal Imagination," 84 Geo. L.J. 301 (1985).

Pastoral Considerations

The Teaching of the Church
Helen Hull Hitchcock

If Christian parents must confront – and answer – the questions addressed in this book, they can no longer invariably count on help from church authorities, or clear and consistent teaching from most churches to support their beliefs. Too often, in fact, church leaders and professionals actively undermine the traditional teachings of their own churches. On homosexuality, as on other key moral issues, clear biblical teaching is often interpreted to mean the opposite of what it says; so homosexuality becomes just one more of the "goods" with which the Creator has endowed his people; practice of a homosexual "lifestyle" is morally neutral, at best, or should be positively endorsed. This view is so deeply entrenched in many churches at the professional level that even clergy who publicly defend the traditional teachings of their own denominations are considered hopelessly "right wing." In this chapter I sketch this often-regrettable story, and set the stage for the two chapters that follow – by Alan Medinger and Fr. John Harvey – which provide reliable pastoral guidance.

I
The Protestant Churches

Nearly every mainline denomination in the United States has been torn by internal strife over proposed (and sometimes adopted) "gay-friendly" anti-discrimination policies. Unlike the Catholic Church, most Protestant denominations in the U.S. are governed by variously named elected legislative bodies who can (and have) literally change(d) church doctrine by ballot. Nearly every core Christian moral teaching has been challenged during the past three decades. Open conflict at the periodic legislative conventions (or synods, or conferences, etc.) has not been rare. Within nearly every mainline Protestant denomination, those who accept traditional Christian moral precepts have been forced into a defensive position by "agents of change" who are most often clergy or full-time church professionals. Even the most fundamental Christian teachings have, thus, become political footballs – to the deep dismay of Christian believers within these denominations. Homosexuality has been at the forefront of these moral and doctrinal issues.

The homosexuality issue has divided United Methodists for several years, particularly after a 1996 statement calling for a change in church doctrine was signed by high-ranking church officials, including fifteen bishops. Methodists were split over the 1998 case of a Nebraska minister who performed a marriage ceremony for two lesbians. The Reverend Jimmy Creech of Omaha was at first acquitted in a church trial by a regional panel of fellow-ministers, but a Council of Bishops panel a few months later ruled that he would not be reappointed as the congregation's pastor.[1]

Although the denomination's prohibition on same-sex unions remains in effect, since the Creech trial more than 1,300 United Methodist ministers said they favor acceptance of homosexual marriage by the church; while an official church poll revealed that 65 percent of church members consider themselves "conservative," and 70 percent believe the Bible is inerrant.[2] The church is the third largest religious body in America, after Catholics and Southern Baptists.

Officials of the Evangelical Lutheran Church in America had the troublesome task of deciding whether to oust one of its pastors in Ames, Iowa, for openly living with his homosexual partner. The ELCA bars "practicing homosexuals" from the ordained ministry. The pastor, Steven Sabin, was married when he was ordained in 1985, and is the father of two daughters, but was divorced five years later.

ELCABishop Philip Hougan said he "reluctantly" brought the charge against Sabin. He is caught, he said, between church teachings and a "sense of compassion for people who feel very excluded or very hurt or denigrated by the church policy." Sabin maintained that church policy violates its own teachings on God's love for all, refused to resign, and said he will not admit to any violation. "Whenever we get the idea that the Gospel is for some and not for others, we are in error. . . . I feel in my very bones that this is my calling right now and I trust in God's time that the church will see the light," said Sabin.[3] Meanwhile, in England, Anglican Archbishop George Carey was pushed from his pulpit during an Easter sermon by demonstrators from a homosexual group called "Outrage!" The archbishop and the Church of England were accused by "Outrage!" of discrimination against homosexuals, in part because Archbishop Carey opposed permitting legalization of teenagers engaging in homosexual practices.[4]

A few months later, at the July 1998 international conference of Anglican bishops, the denomination would vote on the issue of ordaining homosexuals. The negative vote surprised most observers, as a majority of bishops from the UK, Canada, and the U.S. favored changing the church's teaching. The outcome was attributed to the outspoken protest of bishops from Africa.

Similar stories could be recounted about nearly all "mainline" Protestant churches.

While most church members who object to the erosion of church precepts and policies regarding homosexuality have been intimidated into silence, in recent years movements have begun within the mainline denominations to defend traditional Christian teaching on this and other key moral issues, principally abortion. Some of these "renewal" movements, notably in the Methodist and Presbyterian denominations, seem to be growing in influence.

While it will be many years before these grassroots movements can hope to overcome opposition of an entrenched bureaucracy – and a great many clergy – recently there have been some promising signs. In the summer of 2000 their influence was felt at the national governing conferences of United Methodists, Presbyterians and Episcopalians, where proposals to recognize "gay marriages" were eventually defeated – at least for the time being.

II
Catholic Doctrine and Dissent

Catholic doctrine has traditionally been protected by the Church hierarchy, and when challenges to essential teachings become severe and public enough, Church leaders at the highest levels have responded with reaffirmations of the challenged teachings. Despite this relative doctrinal security, however, resistance to these teachings – and to the Church's authority to teach – has not diminished in recent years.

Humanae Vitae, the brief statement of Pope Paul VI issued in 1968 which reaffirmed perennial Christian doctrine about marriage and the meaning of sexual behavior, and that sexual activity must always be open to new human life, precipitated *internal* resistance of historic proportions.

The present papacy has been unique in consistently providing strong social, moral, and dogmatic teaching countering the "counterculture" – from the pope directly, or through letters and statements from curial offices.

Early in his papacy, Pope John Paul II, recognizing the rapidly accelerating decline of moral and religious principles in modern culture, and convinced of the fundamental role of the family in society, established the Pontifical Council for the Family. He also convened a world-wide synod of bishops to address the problems in late September 1980. The Synod on the Family resulted in a key teaching document, *Familiaris Consortio* (The Role of the Christian Family in the Modern World), published a year later. This apostolic letter stresses the "irreplaceable role" of the family in maintaining cultural stability and in transmitting the truth of the faith to future generations. An entire section of this apostolic letter concerns the "Pastoral Care of the Family."

As a further follow-up to the Synod, the Holy See issued the Charter of the Rights of the Family, released by the Pontifical Council on the Family in 1983. The Charter summarizes essential teachings about marriage and family, and Article 5 explicitly upholds the right of parents to expect support and protection from society in the education of their children: "In particular, sex education is a basic right of the parents and must always be carried out under their close supervision, whether at home or in educational centers chosen and controlled by them." Furthermore, "The family has the right to expect that the means of social communication will . . . reinforce the fundamental values of the family," and "the family has the right to be adequately protected, especially with regard to its youngest members, from the negative effects and misuse of the mass media."[5]

This forthright affirmation of core Christian teachings at the highest levels of the Catholic Church has been encouraging to many Christians who are not Catholic as well as a source of authoritative help for Catholics in resisting social pressures contrary to authentic Christian moral principles.

In the 1986 "Letter to the Bishops of the Catholic Church on the Pastoral Care of Homosexual Persons," the Holy See responded to the destructive effect of homosexual activism, and addressed the matter of homosexuality directly and clearly.

However, the Catholic Church, too, suffers greatly from internal divisions, especially the public (and highly publicized) dissent of some of her most influential leaders – theologians, Church officials (both clergy and lay), and regrettably but unsurprisingly, some bishops. Catholics are part of the culture, too, and subject to its influences. The link between homosexuality with other "life and family issues" has become increasingly apparent, notably with abortion, contraception, "sex-ed," and divorce.

Although the American bishops have shown unusual solidarity on abortion (almost no bishop will publicly dispute Church teaching on abortion), homosexual activity is a subject of serious controversy within the Catholic Church. Several recent scandals involving clergy (even bishops) have kept the issue in the media spotlight.

Father Charles Curran achieved national prominence in 1968 when he led a movement among Catholic academics in public dissent from Pope Paul VI's encyclical re-affirming Church doctrine on contraception, *Humanae Vitae*. Curran and his collaborators, although they did not originate moral relativism, firmly implanted into the mainstream of Catholic consciousness the opinion that one need not accept Church teachings one finds unpersuasive.

Usually this individualism was accompanied by a dogmatic instance: that to affirm that something is right or wrong, good or evil, is to be "judgmental." Perhaps the greatest of all sins, according to this view, is to believe that there is such a thing as *personal* sin. And the second greatest is acceptance of any authority ("blind obedience") – in particular, Church authority.

The Curran case left an indelible mark on the Church in America, in part because it showed that authorities, when challenged with open rebellion, usually seem irresolute, disorganized, and ill-prepared for an effective, united response. Thus dissenters, who present a united front in the culture wars, have advanced their agendas virtually unopposed, and have captured the "mainstream": the majority of the Church's influential professional class.

Father Curran, now Professor of Human Values at Southern Methodist University, was the first recipient, in 1992, of New Ways Ministry's "Bridge Building Award," recognizing those who "have promoted discussion, understanding and reconciliation between the lesbian/gay community and the Catholic Church."[6] The citation said that Father Curran "has devoted much energy to addressing the pressing need of the Catholic Church for a viable sexual ethic. He has displayed vision by moving beyond the issues facing single and married individuals to include the crises affecting lesbian and gay persons as well. . . . He has demonstrated courage in developing and articulating a position which he forthrightly acknowledges to be at variance with episcopal [*sic*] teaching."

Father Curran appeared at the first New Ways Ministry Symposium in 1981 and "spoke about the ethics of a same-sex relationship. This action, we are convinced," says NWM, "did not gain him favor from the Congregation for the Doctrine of the Faith." NWM is thankful for Father Curran's "theological and strategic advice . . . most notably to our co-founders, [Sister] Jeannine Gramick and [Father] Robert Nugent, who have encountered similar difficulties with Church authorities."

Sister Jeannine Gramick, of the School Sisters of Notre Dame, and Father Robert Nugent, of the Society of the Divine Savior, founded New Ways Ministry in 1977, originally under the auspices of the leftist Quixote Center in Maryland. NWM and its co-founders have been under investigation by the Vatican for at least fifteen years.

Their "gay and lesbian" advocacy activities drew the attention of the archbishop of Washington, DC, James Hickey (now Cardinal Hickey), who banned them from appearing in his archdiocese. By 1984, early investigation of the activities of NWM led the Holy See to require the founders to separate themselves from leadership of their organization.

Cardinal Adam Maida of Detroit headed a commission that began its investigations in 1988, and presented its results at a meeting in Rome with Sister Gramick and Father Nugent in July 1994.[7] It would be five years before a decision was made. Meanwhile, the NWM founders established the Catholic Parents Network, "an association of Catholic parents of gay and lesbian children for support and resources," according to its advertising flyer. And New Ways Ministry continued as before.

A bishop was NWM's 1995 "Bridge Building" recipient. Bishop Thomas Gumbleton, auxiliary bishop of Detroit since 1968, "was an early voice against discrimination toward lesbian/gay people," said NWM's award citation to the Bishop. In 1974, the citation said, when a man was fired from the Detroit archdiocesan newspaper for being "gay" and went on a hunger strike, "Bishop Gumbleton, along with Bishop Joseph Imesch, called on the Church of Detroit to recognize its 'serious obligation to root out structures and attitudes that discriminate against the homosexual as a person,' and pledged to 'exert our leadership on behalf of this effort.'"[8]

In an address to a Call to Action conference in November 1997, Bishop Gumbleton stressed that homosexuals have a right to follow their own consciences "and the rest of us have no right to make any judgments," that not all homosexuals are "called to the 'charism of celibacy,'" and suggested some form of ceremony blessing homosexual partnerships.[9]

At a New Ways Ministry Symposium in Pittsburgh in March 1997, Bishop Gumbleton urged all homosexuals, including priests, to "come out," "because that is how our church is going to truly change." The meeting drew 650 people, nearly half of them priests and religious.[10]

The following quotation is featured prominently on the home page of the Internet web site, *Theology Library – Gay and Lesbian Catholicism*:

> If you say someone is disordered, that means there is something wrong with that person at the root of their being. I can't believe God would make someone who is wrong from the very beginning. – Most Rev. Thomas Gumbleton, auxiliary bishop of Detroit

These statements, and similar comments which appear in nearly all Catholic homosexual-rights propaganda ("God loves us, too," "God loves gay and lesbian people") work much like the old chestnut, "When did you stop beating your wife?" By making acceptance of the entire spectrum of the homosexualist agenda a matter of "love," the homosexual rights lobby has created an effective taboo. Nobody can say anything negative about any aspect of homosexuality or homosexualist activism without paying the penalty of being judged "unloving" and "homophobic." This stratagem has worked very well.

Such statements are useful, too, to "prove" the homosexualists' key argument: (1) homosexuality is a "God-given" aspect of one's nature; (2) sexual (genital) expression is natural and essential to one's well-being; (3) *ergo*, God intends homosexuals to engage in sex acts; (4) *ergo*, any religion or any person who maintains that homosexuality is *not* natural but is an acquired disorder which may be prevented or even cured, that God intends the use of human sexuality to be exclusively within marriage for the union of man and woman and for the establishment of families, is *anathema*. Hence the urgent determination to "reform" the doctrine of the Catholic Church.

Francis DeBernardo, executive director of New Ways Ministry, said in a statement at a Religious Leadership Roundtable Press Conference July 24, 1998,

> As early as 1975 . . . the Vatican proclaimed that the [homosexual] orientation was "innate," not some-

thing chosen or acquired. Since that time, Catholic leaders and people in the pews have begun to embrace gay and lesbian people, fight for their rights, and welcome them into their communities. They have recognized that gay and lesbian people were created by God. Thirty dioceses have begun pastoral outreach programs for lesbian and gay people, and new initiatives are begun in parishes each week.[11]

Although some bishops have misgivings about such "pastoral outreach" programs, and some have forbidden Dignity and New Ways Ministry to conduct programs in their dioceses, many others tolerate them, and some have positively fostered these "initiatives" within their dioceses, in particular, the National Association of Catholic Diocesan Gay and Lesbian Ministries, whose objectives differ negligibly from those of Dignity and NWM, and which works to establish diocesan offices and programs for "outreach" to homosexuals.

Bishop Keith Symons of Palm Beach issued a statement in May 1997 permitting a "retreat for parents of gay/lesbian sons/daughters" presented by Father Nugent and Sister Gramick. As reported by the NACDGLM News, the bishop said that he would not cancel the program "despite protests by a few well-intentioned but ill-informed persons," because "I have consulted fellow bishops of dioceses where they have spoken" and "am assured that Father Nugent and Sister Gramick present the authentic teaching of the Catholic Church with compassionate ministry outreach in conformity with Sacred Scripture."[12]

Bishop Symons was forced to resign in June 1998, for having molested five boys.

A year later, Bishop Patrick Ziemann of Santa Rosa, California, resigned after his homosexual "lover," a man whom the bishop had ordained to the priesthood, filed a lawsuit accusing Ziemann of sexual assault. A former auxiliary bishop of Los Angeles, Ziemann had served as bishop of Santa Rosa since 1993. His seven-year incumbency had been marked by sexual scandals. At the time of his resignation July 21, 1999, Ziemann was chairman of two important committees of the U.S. bishops' conference, the Committee on the Laity and the Subcommittee on Catechesis, among other conference offices.

This internal dissent and – worse – scandal in the Catholic Church is not only debilitating to those who are faithful to Church teachings and confusing to nearly everyone, but the apparent ambiguity within the episcopacy itself also provides a convenient blind behind which too many clergy take cover when they face conflict and are forced to address the issue.

For example, a Seattle pastor, having succumbed to legal pressure brought by victims, announced to his congregation at Sunday Mass that his curate is a pedophile, but enjoined his parishioners to overlook the priest's criminally abusive behavior: "Because there's a small area of his life that's dysfunctional, I don't think you should take away his opportunity to give his gifts to others."[13]

Other priests, encouraged by activist groups, are praised when they reveal their homosexuality publicly. A priest from the diocese of Grand Rapids "got lots of hugs" after he told his parishioners that he is "gay." "I was just filled with tears, there were so many hugs," said Father Martin Kurylowicz. "It means more now, because they know the real me." The priest said he spoke up after attending a national conference on gay issues sponsored by New Ways Ministry in March 1997.

His bishop was "extremely supportive," Father Kurylowicz said. Bishop Robert Rose told a reporter for *The Grand Rapids Press* that he believes the priest's views on homosexuality are in line with Church teaching, but he will "be watching to see what the reaction of his people is and if there is any other response from people around the diocese."[14]

A shocking and controversial "special report" on homosexuality in the Catholic priesthood that appeared in the *Kansas City Star* is still reverberating. These reports said that studies showed that priests are dying of AIDS at a rate at least four times that of the general U.S. population. This claim was later challenged, but no one disputed the problem of homosexual clergy. Bishop Raymond Boland of Kansas City, Missouri, was quoted in the opening story in the series:

In an earlier interview, Bishop Raymond J. Boland of the Diocese of Kansas City-St. Joseph said the AIDS deaths show that priests are human.

"Much as we would regret it, it shows that human nature is human nature," Boland said. "And all of us are heirs to all of the misfortunes that can be foisted upon the human race." Boland thinks Church leaders now are doing a better job.

"I do feel today that a lot of our men get many opportunities – the standard of spiritual direction, the standard of formation is much higher," Boland said. "And in all of the seminaries, we have people who are trained counselors."[15]

Bishop Boland's comments did little to assuage the growing uneasiness of faithful Catholic families, who are concerned about the "vocations crisis" and take very seriously the call of Church authorities to encourage their sons to consider a priestly vocation; but who also fear what these young men might encounter if do go into the seminary or a religious order. Nor was Catholic parents' concern diminished by a book on homosexuality among Catholic clergy, *The Changing Face of the Priesthood*, by Father Donald B. Cozzens, president and rector of the diocese of Cleveland's St. Mary Seminary and Graduate School of Theology. Father Cozzens also has a doctorate in psychology. "Considering Orientation" is the chapter in which the author claims that there is a disproportionate number of homosexuals in the priesthood – and wrote that "the priesthood is rapidly becoming a gay profession."[16]

In a review of Cozzens' book, Tom Fox of the liberal *National Catholic Reporter,* said that whether the priesthood is a "gay profession"

. . . is a devilishly difficult question to ask, first because almost no one in the hierarchical ranks wants anything to do with it, and because one can only approach it through a minefield planted wide with homophobes, right-wing zealots who see homosexu-

al clergy as a particularly noxious manifestation of a
liberal agenda, and the Church's teaching that the
homosexual orientation is "objectively disordered."

Curiously, although Father Cozzens says that most priests
who are sexual abusers target teenage boys while most other child
molesters target girls, he believes mandatory celibacy is the problem: "To insist that there is simply no correlation between mandatory celibacy and the present crisis over clergy misconduct with
minors looks like bureaucratic bullying as long as the Vatican
remains opposed to even discussion concerning the systems
undergirding the priestly lifestyle."

In an interview with Aaron Brown of ABC News, Father
Cozzens said that he had "a little knot in the pit of my stomach as
I wrote that [the priesthood is becoming a "gay profession"], but
it's my experience, and it has been supported by a number of other
priests to date that I know that have a lot of pastoral experience,
and many of them have seminary experience."

Did he have recommendations for the renewal and transformation of the priesthood?

"Once we have some . . . honest conversations, I think we're
going to be moving in the right direction. Will there be optional
celibacy? Personally I think there will be. I don't know how soon.
I think that will be a factor that is positive. But . . . I don't have a
program, a personal program for the renewal of the priesthood."[17]

Meanwhile, the saga of Father Nugent and Sister Gramick continued through the "Jubilee Year," primarily because they had
largely ignored a Vatican "Notification" in 1999 to cease their
"pastoral ministry" with homosexuals, which had continued
uninterrupted during the years following the 1994 Maida commission report.

In the summer of 1999, five years after the Maida commission
report had found "serious deficiencies in their writings and pastoral activities which were incompatible with the fullness of
Christian morality," and more than a decade after the commission's investigation began, the Congregation for the Doctrine of
the Faith issued a directive permanently prohibiting both Nugent

and Gramick from "any pastoral work involving homosexual persons," citing "ambiguities and errors" and serious deficiencies in their writings and pastoral activities, which were incompatible with the fullness of Christian morality. The July 13, 1999, *Notification* from the CDF, approved by Pope John Paul II, also prohibited the pair from holding any office in their respective religious orders.

Bishop Joseph Fiorenza, president of the NCCB, in a July 13 statement announcing the Vatican action, said that the "Congregation was obliged to act on account of these deficiencies," but stressed that the bishops "heard the call to offer Gospel-based pastoral assistance" to homosexuals in issuing *Always Our Children*, condemned "violent malice in speech or in action" against homosexuals and strongly emphasized that "those with homosexual inclinations deserve our care and respect."[18]

Father Nugent said he accepted the Holy See's decision, while Sister Gramick complained of "oppression." She issued a statement refusing to obey the Vatican directive. Although she had said in 1994 that she had been "extremely pleased with the way the commission conducted itself" (the pair had even been permitted to correct the minutes of the proceedings),[19] her September 23, 1999, statement said that the "composition of the [Maida] commission . . . resulted in imbalance and bias." She said that on reflection, she was "so overwhelmed by the authoritarian methods that I could not see the justice of God in the outcome."[20]

Both continued giving lectures, however, and complaints about the Vatican's decision became their usual subject.

Criticism of the Vatican among their supporters reached such a pitch that in November, 1999 Bishop Fiorenza issued a news release, pointing out that

> . . . evaluations of their programs and writings over many years have indicated that neither Sister Gramick nor Father Nugent fully reflect the constant teaching of the Church that homosexual activity is intrinsically disordered. The Congregation for the Doctrine of the Faith has the responsibility to see that

those who exercise pastoral ministry and teach in the name of the Church do so fully and accurately. The Congregation gave both Sister Gramick and Father Nugent several opportunities to express the belief of the Church which unfortunately they did not do satisfactorily. As a result the Congregation had no alternative but to take action. I am glad that both Sister Gramick and Father Nugent continue to follow the way of the Church by accepting the judgment of the Congregation.[21]

Bishop Fiorenza issued a more detailed statement on November 17. He said the bishops "deplore as a horrible evil any malice in speech or action against homosexual persons and call upon all who engage in such acts to repent of their behavior," but he responded to some of the critics of the Holy See's Notification, mentioning in particular *Is Homosexuality a Sin?* a booklet co-authored by Nugent and Gramick, published by PFLAG, which contained "misstatements" about Church teaching. The bishop's statement said that "the *Notification* cannot be used to claim that the Church teaches that persons of homosexual inclination are intrinsically evil persons." It clarified that "it is not an invasion of conscience for the Church to ask those who minister in Her name about their adherence to Church teaching," it defended the authority of Church ("It is the obligation of the Holy See to ensure that all who hold offices in religious communities adhere to the fullness of the faith, without reservation"), and it noted that the Holy Father "is the ultimate superior of all members of religious institutes."

The decision of Sister Gramick and Father Nugent to abide by the decision of the Holy See is laudable. I want to urge them again, in the spirit of filial obedience to the supreme authority of the Church, to reflect more intensely and prayerfully on the Church's authentic teaching and ask the Holy Spirit to guide their minds and hearts to embrace this truth unambiguously.[22]

But they did not do so. In May they were summoned to Rome to meet with Vatican officials from the CDF and the Congregation for Institutes of Consecrated Life – and with the superiors of their religious orders, the Society of the Divine Savior and the School Sisters of Notre Dame.

In a short statement on May 30, Father Nugent accepted the terms of the *Notification*. However, Sister Gramick refused. After her meeting on May 24 with Sister Rosemary Howarth, the Superior General of the School Sisters of Notre Dame, where she was called to obedience to the Notification and to her own provincial's orders to "a new ministry of full-time study," Sister Gramick announced that she would not comply. In a statement on May 25, she likened herself to a battered woman who "has found sufficient strength to name the oppression . . . she is often pursued by the batterer, who tries to cower her into submission and begin the cycle of intimidation once again." She again complained about the Holy See's injustices; "after finding my voice to tell my story, I choose not to collaborate in my own oppression," she said.[23]

Sister Gramick has not yet been expelled from her order. Her cause is being strenuously advanced by prominent feminist activists. Loretto Sister Maureen Fiedler of "Catholics Speak Out" (at the Quixote Center, where New Ways Ministry originated) urged a letter writing campaign to save Sister Gramick from dismissal. Sister Joan Chittister, a Benedictine from Erie, Pennsylvania, and feminist theologian Rosemary Ruether used their regular columns in the *National Catholic Reporter* to decry the "oppressive patriarchy" that disciplined Sister Gramick.[24] A collection of documentation on the Nugent-Gramick case is featured on the website of the NCR.

III
"Culture of Death" or the "Civilization of Love"

Pope John Paul II has repeatedly stressed the fundamental interconnection of "life issues" and the duty of laity to be able to "explain and defend certain fundamental truths and values essential to society's well-being, especially in relation to the inalienable dignity and value of human life and its transmission in a stable family setting," and to "promote legislation which corresponds to the moral law and to seek to reform." Or, as Jesuit theologian Donald Keefe has expressed it, "Moral decay is the indispensable prelude to conversion to the new religion, which is inevitably an idolatrous imaging of a false god. The Catholic imaging is nuptial; the idolatrous, homosexual. It is by no means happenstance that the classic pagan cultures were infested with homosexuality."[25] In his 1993 *Ad limina* address to bishops of New York and Pennsylvania the Pope urged bishops "to increase your efforts to restore respect for God's wise and loving plan for human sexuality"; and "when necessary, you must take the 'appropriate measures to ensure that the faithful are guarded from every doctrine and theory contrary to it' [*Veritatis Splendor* §116]." He told the bishops that "[y]our priests should be helped to give their firm assent to this teaching and to commit themselves to forming the consciences of those entrusted to their pastoral care according to the full truth of the Gospel."[26]

In his address to the bishops of Ireland in June 1999, Pope John Paul II again drew attention to the pervasive corrosion of moral sense in our time:

> It is also true that the exaggerated individualism which sometimes accompanies increased material prosperity has brought in its wake a declining sense of God's presence and of the transcendent meaning of human life. The relativism which then takes hold often leads to a rejection of the objective foundations of morality and an overly subjective understanding of conscience. . . . There follows a corrosion of the sense that Christianity teaches the truth – a truth which we ourselves have not devised but which comes to us as gift. This can in turn lead to discouragement and to the belief that the Church no longer has anything of relevance to say to the men and women of our day. But in fact Christian experience over the centuries, and in our own time also, shows that faith, when tested, can emerge stronger, freer and more vigorous, just

as the history of the Church in Ireland eloquently testifies.[27]

In this message, the Pope calls on bishops to "proclaim the truth courageously, even if what you teach sometimes goes against socially accepted opinion," and that this "must be his constant concern to ensure that the true content of Catholic doctrine is taught effectively, [for] nothing can substitute for the power of the truths of the faith themselves to attract, convince and transform a person's inner experience."[28] (He specifically addressed the scandal of sexual abuse by clergy in this message.)

The Holy Father also said that because of the weak "sense of sin," bishops need to place particular emphasis on the Sacrament of Penance:

> Prevailing trends in contemporary culture weaken the sense of sin, particularly because of a diminished consciousness of God who is all holy and calls his people to holiness of life. A great pastoral effort is therefore required in order to help the faithful to recover the sense of what sin is in relation to God, and consequently to have a profound appreciation of the beauty and joy of the Sacrament of Penance. This requires emphasis on the Sacrament in diocesan pastoral programs and Jubilee initiatives, calling Catholics to encounter anew the uniquely transforming experience that is individual, integral confession and absolution. The personal nature of sin, conversion, forgiveness and reconciliation is the reason why personal confession of sins and individual absolution are required (cf. *Catechism of the Catholic Church*, 1484).[29]

During a June 1999 visit to his homeland, Pope John Paul II reminded the Polish parliament that "Even pluralist states cannot abandon ethical norms in public life," and he quotes his encyclical *Veritatis Splendor* concerning the "risk of an alliance between democracy and ethical relativism, which would remove any sure moral reference point from political and social life, and on a deeper level make the acknowledgment of truth impossible. Indeed 'if there is no ultimate truth to guide and direct political activity, then ideas and convictions can easily be manipulated for reasons of power. As history demonstrates, a democracy without values easily turns into open or thinly disguised totalitarianism'" (*VS*, No. 101).[30]

In his 1994 *Letter to Families* the Pope contrasted the "Culture of Death," the society in which we now live, with the "Civilization of Love" to which we must aspire. He observes that the destructive effects of utilitarian attitudes which regard people as objects of use are widespread. "To be convinced that this is the case," he writes, "one need only look at certain sexual education programs introduced into the schools" even when parents protest.

> Who can deny that our age is one marked by a great crisis, which appears above all as a profound 'crisis of truth'? A crisis of truth means . . . a crisis of concepts. Do the words love, freedom, sincere gift and even person and rights of the person really convey their essential meaning? . . . Only if the truth about freedom and the communion of persons in marriage and in the family can regain its splendor will the building of a civilization of love truly begin and will it then be possible to speak concretely . . . about promoting the dignity of marriage and the family.[31]

Conclusion

As the family goes, so goes the world. Now more than ever, the Catholic Church is a "sign of contradiction" to the world and a stumbling block to the culture of our time. But who will heed the words of the Holy Father and the moral precepts of the Church?

Can we rebuild the collapsing social institutions of the culture? Can we find a way to help the Rachels and Alans who have been abandoned not only by their husbands and fathers but by the schools and churches and leaders they depend upon? Who can now give parents like Rachel encouragement and reliable support in her care and concern for the child entrusted to her? Who should have helped provide guidance and protection for Alan and his peers? Why didn't they do it?

Where are our leaders who may help repair the crumbling moral structure of our world? Or is it too late to prevent "calamity and disaster"?

What can we do? Can we help these families in trouble, heal the broken hearts of parents and the emotional anguish of their afflicted children? Can we relieve their suffering?

Endnotes

1. "Minister in Lesbian Ceremony to Be Ousted," Associated Press, May 7, 1998 (from New York Times web site.)

2. Mark Tooley, Institute for Religion and Democracy, "United Methodists Are Plagued by Division," United Press International Radio Commentary, May 15, 1998.

3. Mary Neubauer, "Admitting Homosexuality," Associated Press, January 31, 1998.

4. "Homosexual activists seize Pulpit from Archbishop Carey," Religion Today/GC Internet news service, April 14, 1998.

5. Cf. *Charter of the Rights of the Family*, 1983. Article 5.

6. "Bridge Building Awards" quotations all appeared on the New Ways Ministry web page, November 25, 1997 (NWM web address in July 99: www.us.netlepf/NEWWAYS.htm). There are dozens of homosexual advocacy sites on the Internet, several of them "Catholic."

7. Other NWM investigative commission members were Bishop John Snyder of St. Augustine, then chairman of the NCCB Committee on Women; Dr. Janet Smith, philosophy professor at the University of Dallas and author of *Humanae Vitae A Generation Later*, and Monsignor James J. Mulligan, Director of Priestly Life and Ministry office of the diocese of Allentown, Pennsylvania.

8. Both were then auxiliary bishops of Detroit. Bishop Imesch was made bishop of Joliet, Illinois in 1979.

9. Robert Delaney, "Bishop Says Church Should Improve Ministry to Gays," Catholic News Service, November 24, 1997.

10. Tom Roberts, "Bishop Wants Clergy and Laity Out of the Closet," *National Catholic Reporter*, March 21, 1997.

Helen Hull Hitchcock

11. Francis DeBernardo, July 28, 1998, statement to National Religious Leadership Roundtable, from New Ways Ministry web site (www.us.net/epf/NEWWAYS.HTM), July 8, 1999.

12. "Bishop Symons Allows Retreat for Parents," NACDGLM News, August 1997, p. 4.

13. Jason Berry, *Lead us Not Into Temptation*, 1992 Doubleday, p. 331.

14. Charles Honey, "Gay Priest 'Comes Out' after New Ways Symposium," *The Grand Rapids Press*, March 29, 1997 (reprinted on the New Ways Ministry web page, November 1997).

15. Judy L. Thomas, "Special report: AIDS in the Priesthood," *The Kansas City Star*, January 29, 2000.

16. Donald B. Cozzens, *The Changing Face of the Priesthood*. February 2000. Collegeville, Ill.: Liturgical Press.

17. Aaron Brown, "Priestly Ponderings," interview with Father Cozzens. ABC News.com, July 2, 2000.

18. Bishop Joseph A. Fiorenza, "Statement on Notification," June 13, 1999.

19. *National Catholic Reporter*, October 14, 1994, p 6.

20. Statement of Jeannine Gramick, SSND, Regarding Discernment on the Notification of the Congregation for the Doctrine of the Faith," September 23, 1999. (from website of the *National Catholic Reporter:* www.natcath.org. The *NCR* web site prominently features a collection of articles and documents on the Nugent and Gramick case in August 2000.)

21. Bishop Joseph Fiorenza, News Release from NCCB Department of Communications, November 15, 1999.

22. Bishop Joseph Fiorenza, statement regarding the Sister Gramick and Father Nugent Notification, November 17, 1999.

23. Statement of Sister Jeannine Gramick, May 25, 2000.

24. Joan Chittister, "Of force, fear: It takes courage to stand up to leaders who punish in name of the Gospel," *NCR* August 11, 2000, p 18; Rosemary Ruether, "Renewed in zone of truth: To overcome 'structures of deceit,' refuse to collaborate with them," *NCR* August 25, 2000, p. 16.

25. Donald Keefe, S.J., private letter to this writer, July 2, 1998. Father Keefe was Professor of Systematic Theology at St. John's Seminary, Dunwoodie, the New York Archdiocesan Seminary, and author of *Covenantal Theology*.

26. Pope John Paul II, *Ad Limina* Message to New Jersey and Pennsylvania bishops, November 11, 1993, §3-6. *Origins,* December 23, 1993, p. 485.

27. Pope John Paul II, *Ad limina* Message to Irish bishops, June 26, 1999, §2

28. Ibid. §4

29. Ibid. §8

30. Pope John Paul II, Message to Polish Parliament, June 1, 1999, §5

31. Pope John Paul II, *Letter to Families,* February 22, 1994, §13, "The two civilizations."

Calling Oneself "Gay" or "Lesbian" Clouds One's Self-Perception

Alan P. Medinger

In the weeks after Thanksgiving and Christmas, the calls always come in: anguished parents telling us that their son or daughter had just announced to them that he or she is gay or lesbian. "Last night my son told his father and me that he is gay. What do we do?" For twenty years I have been Director of Regeneration, a Christian ministry for men and women seeking to overcome homosexuality. We also work with family members of homosexual people. Far and away the most hurting people we minister to are Christian parents who have just found out about their child's homosexuality.

There is a reason why we get an increase in the number of these calls after the Thanksgiving and Christmas holidays. Typically, the son or daughter just went off to college in the fall. At college, for the first time, he or she encountered a sizeable and active community of homosexual people. These sons and daughters had, no doubt, struggled with homosexual feelings for a number of years; some had been homosexually active. But their homosexuality had been kept under wraps. They sensed that something was wrong with it. They certainly didn't want their parents or siblings or the broader community to know that they were "queer." They lived in isolation and shame with their problem.

Then, at college, they were able to speak with gays who were open and free with their homosexuality. These people were not ashamed. They were gay and lesbian, and they were proud of it. The son or daughter was told, "Don't fight it; this is who you are. Your unhappiness is not because you are gay, but because of your false shame and your need to repress who you are." The argument for "coming out" is powerful and convincing. Finally, the son or daughter has found a community that understands them. These are their people. Very quickly the son or daughter identifies with the group, buying into the belief that openness about "who they are" brings self-acceptance and freedom.

So, on the first visit back home, which is often around Thanksgiving or Christmas, comes the message, "Mom, Dad, I'm gay," or "Mom, I'm a lesbian." Hence, the calls that we get after the holidays.

Sadly, the scenario I just described is occurring more and more frequently well before college. The media's positive portrayal of homosexuality, the nature of sex education and diversity training being offered in schools, and the ubiquitous propaganda by a powerful gay community are all combining to lead children to declare at a younger and younger age that, "I am gay!"

Whether this declaration is made at fourteen or twenty-two or forty-two, it is always indicative of one thing: the individual has embraced a false identity. An understanding of this truth can have tremendous significance in the lives of men and women who find themselves with homosexual attractions – and to their parents and loved ones.

Before going on, let me describe how I will be using certain words. Because there has been a shift over the years in the way that the word "homosexual" is used, and because the use of "gay" with respect to homosexuality is of fairly recent origin, and most of all, because these words have been used intentionally in ways that will promote people's acceptance of homosexuality, some simple clarifications are in order. I will avoid using "homosexual" as a noun. Doing so immediately makes it an identity as in "he is a homosexual." I will use it as an adjective or as a verb object such as "a homosexual person" or "he is homosexual." "Homosexual" will be used to describe the condition wherein one's primary sexual and romantic attractions are toward people of the same sex, a condition that is *primarily* involuntary. I will use it for both men and women. I will use "gay" with respect to the identity that a person *willingly* takes on when he or she decides to view life through the prism of his or her homosexuality, and when the person casts his or her lot with a certain sub-culture. Dr. Joseph Nicolosi's explanations in this area have been very helpful, especially when he speaks of the "non-gay homosexual" person, the person who has homosexual feelings, but has not let that define who he or she is. Gay people are inconsistent as to whether gay applies to men alone, or to men and women. I will use it to apply to both.

Who You Are or What You Do?

Now, suppose that the Thanksgiving holiday message was not the son's declaration, "I'm gay," but, "Mom and Dad, Mike and I have been having sex together." Would it make a difference? It might at first. Parents, being what they are, would likely grab onto any hope that this was just some sort of temporary aberrational behavior, some state of confusion or a phase that wouldn't last. Maybe loneliness or insecurity caused him to do something he never would have done otherwise. Maybe their fairly naïve son was seduced by a gay student.

Although the parents might try to grasp at these or other explanations, quite likely at the same time they are harboring a deeper fear, "My son is gay." So much has our culture shifted the concept of homosexuality from what someone *does* to what someone *is*, that even the most hopeful parent will have difficulty separating the two. So effectively have those who think that homosexuality is acceptable promoted the concept of homosexuality as being an identity, that all of us, even those who have seen the error in this kind of thinking, have to keep reminding ourselves to separate what a person does from who he or she is.

Of course for the son or daughter it makes a huge difference. For them the distinction is intensely personal. We all have a powerful desire to justify ourselves, to feel good about ourselves, and "being" is neutral, whereas "doing" can be wrong or sinful. Especially for people with low self-esteem – a very common characteristic among homosexual people – shifting the focus from what I do to who I am can take a person from the realm of condemnation to a world of acceptance. And, once the son or daughter has made "gay" or "lesbian" their identity, they are quite likely to move on to accept a whole group of corollaries that will further strengthen this self-perception:

1. I must have been born this way.
2. If I was born that way, God made me this way.
3. If God made me this way, how can there be anything wrong with it?
4. It is my nature, and I must be true to my nature.
5. If it's my nature, I can't change.
6. If I try to change, I would be trying to go against my nature, and that would be
harmful.
7. Accepting myself as gay feels so good – I feel like a thousand pound load has been lifted off my back – so it must be okay.
8. If people can't accept my being gay, something is wrong with them.
9. If people can't accept my being gay, then they don't accept me, because that's who I am.

Taken together these statements simply cannot stand up against logic or against Church teaching. They are all false, but that is to be expected; they are all based on a false premise – homosexuality is an identity.

It does make a huge difference whether the person who feels homosexual attractions, or is active homosexually, does or does not take on a homosexual or gay or lesbian identity. And, because it makes a huge difference to the individual, it also should matter greatly to their friends and loved ones, to society and to the Church. How we deal with the homosexually oriented person, and how society and the Church deal with homosexuality, will depend significantly on whether or not we accept the homosexual *identity*.

A False Identity

Let's carry our Thanksgiving holiday scenario a little further. The daughter says, "Mom and Dad, I'm a lesbian." Dad asks, "What makes you think you are a lesbian?" The daughter responds, "Because I'm sexually and emotionally attracted to women and not to men." Mom then asks, "Why do you think you are sexually and emotionally attracted to women?" The daughter replies, "Because I'm a lesbian."

Such circular thinking sounds absurd, but it is actually where we are in our understanding of being homosexual today. No one has been able to identify a homosexual person by any criteria other than by their behavior and sexual attractions.

This is similar to an experience I had when I went to an ophthalmologist about a chronic bloodshot eye. He carefully examined my eye and told me I had conjunctivitis. I asked what that meant, and he said, "It means that your eye is bloodshot." I said, "Thank you very much," paid my bill and left – a little poorer and no wiser.

Researchers have been trying for years to determine the cause of homosexuality. In effect, what they are trying to do is to identify some characteristic that makes homosexually attracted people different from heterosexually attracted people. As Dr. Satinover points out,[1] their efforts have come to naught. None of the studies, so highly touted in the media as proving a genetic cause for homosexuality, has been replicated in further studies. I might point out also that most of these studies have been by researchers who themselves are homosexually oriented. This itself certainly does not discredit their research, but one has to wonder why the other 95–97 percent of researchers don't come up with similar findings. It may just point to how much gays want to believe that the condition is who they are.

The concept of a homosexual person is quite recent. Even the word "homosexual" was a nineteenth-century creation, developed with the emergence of psychiatry. For millennia mankind had recognized homosexual behavior, but saw it as just that – a behavior engaged in by some people. And although some people were clearly observed as engaging in frequent and exclusive homosexual behavior, no need was found to see these people as different in any way but their behavior.[2]

Looked at historically, the gay identity seems to have come about as a defensive measure, a means of giving legitimacy to certain feelings and behaviors. The formation of the gay sub-culture and its associated political movement over the past thirty years has been largely an effort to give an identity to people who feel same-sex attractions. In this respect, the gay identity is part of a political strategy, used by gay leaders to do what political people have always done: expand their power and influence by convincing people to identify more and more strongly with their group. An "us-them" attitude, a powerful sense of victimhood, and a sense of superiority empower the gay movement and expand the concept of being a homosexual person to the point at which viewing the world from any other perspective becomes almost impossible.

The truth is, however, until someone can come up with a description for homosexuality that goes beyond merely describing the direction of a person's sexual and romantic attractions, our using "homosexual" as an identity obscures truth and sows seeds of confusion.

The Seductive Power of Being 'Gay'

When, in 1979, I finally gave up and surrendered my life to Jesus Christ in a prayer meeting in the basement of a Catholic parish school near Baltimore, the changes in me were so profound that for weeks I wanted to run around with my hands up in the air shouting, "I'm free; I'm free at last!" A glorious manifestation of this freedom was that the power of homosexuality had been lifted from me. The power that had driven me for so many years had been broken, and now I was free to start living a new life as the man I knew God had created me to be.

Ironically, a similar feeling of freedom often comes over a young person when he or she first declares, "I am gay," or "I am a lesbian." Finally, there is self-acceptance, an end to self-condemnation and perhaps – at least among those who understand – an end of the condemnation by others.

Even in today's permissive culture, growing up with a homosexual orientation is not an easy thing for a young person. The first feeling that such a child experiences is not that "I am gay," but rather that "I am different," and different always translates into *less than.* "I can't do what other boys (girls) do. I don't measure up." Words like "queer" or "fag" or "dyke" are heard. "The

Church teaches that the things that I long to do are grievous sins. I dare not tell my parents or friends what is going on inside." Many start to lead double lives, outwardly acting like their peers, but on the inside feeling entirely estranged from them. Internal doubts and emotional isolation lead to strong feelings of self-condemnation.

Then comes the message, "This is who you truly are. You are not a pervert, some sort of reprobate, a fairy or a queer; you are gay, you are a lesbian. You don't have to pretend anymore. There is nothing wrong with who you are. You can shed your shame and walk freely as the gay person you are!"

How powerful. How heady. This person does feel free at last, but tragically, this new-found freedom will lead this young person down roads he or she had never anticipated, roads that lead to anything but freedom.

Does It Matter?

Is this just an argument over terms, or does it matter whether we use homosexuality as a behavior or as an identity? I maintain that it matters a great deal – especially for the homosexually oriented man or woman. How a homosexual person views his or her homosexuality not only determines their current identity, it can in large part determine that person's future. When a woman decides that she is a lesbian, or when a man decides that he is a gay, a number of things happen:

1. *Other beliefs about homosexuality become accepted and enforced.* The nine corollaries that I offered earlier take root in the person, and he or she gains a vested interest in their being true. Gay militancy is not just about ending discrimination against homosexual people; it is a demand that society embrace these nine beliefs about homosexuality. When "homosexual" is who I am, then it is true that if you reject my homosexuality, you reject me. The idea, "hate the sin, and love the sinner" is an anathema to many gays because they have identified themselves as the sin. This is a stumbling block between many parents and their homosexual sons and daughters. An impasse arises because the Christian parents cannot in conscience say that their child's homosexuality is good, while

the child has so much invested in being gay or lesbian that the parents' disapproval of the child's lifestyle is seen as a rejection of him or her.

2. *Life becomes limited and narrowed.* Look in a directory of gay organizations in any large city, and you may be astounded at how many gay organizations there are. You can join an organization for gay Catholics, gay Episcopalians, even gay Mormons. You can be a member of the gay medical or gay bar associations. You can join gay AA or play in a gay volleyball or bowling league. You can even be a gay Republican. So much have some people allowed their sexual attractions to define them, that their relationships and activities become overwhelmingly influenced by this identity. This personal identity becomes merged into an identity with a certain group of people. Implied in all of this is the attitude that no one can understand them but another gay person, and so to varying extents they cut off the other 95–97 percent of humanity.

3. *Obedience to the Church's teaching is made more difficult.* Problems here can take several forms. An individual who believes that the Church probably is technically correct in saying that homosexual practice is sinful may drift to the position of some theologians, saying in effect that homosexuality may not be God's desire for us, but given the reality of one's "homosexual nature," all a person can do is try and be the best homosexual possible. Usually, this means finding one partner and becoming faithful to that person. Some recommend this even though they know that for homosexually oriented men monogamy is close to impossible.[3]

Some may accept the Church's teaching that homosexual behavior is sinful but take a "cheap grace" attitude to it. I'm gay, that's who I am; God understands this, so he'll forgive me. The spiritual danger in this should be obvious. It denies the terrible power of sin, and it demeans the price that our Lord paid that we might be forgiven our sins. It is one thing to seek to be obedient and fail; it is quite another to presume upon God's grace, actually using grace as an excuse to sin.

Others may simply reject the Church's teaching. If the number of people who are members of Dignity (which affirms homosexuality) versus the number in Courage (which helps homosexual

Catholics to live in obedience to Church teaching) is reflective of homosexual Catholics in general, it would appear that a significant majority of homosexual Catholics have concluded that they can remain Catholic and reject the Church's teaching on homosexuality. Were homosexuality seen as merely a matter of behavior, this would be harder to pull off. The Church has always been called to tell us that certain behaviors (that we found attractive) are against God's will. But when the Church is trying to tell me that I cannot live according to my nature, then obviously the Church is wrong. Hopefully, it will one day catch up with the times.

On the other side, people who see their homosexual attractions as primarily bent toward a specific form of sexual sin will see their struggles as being in common with the struggles of all Christian people who have within them a powerful propensity to satisfy certain immediate desires in ways that God has ruled off-limits. True, the heterosexually oriented person has the prospect of one day experiencing a fulfilling sexual life in marriage, and homosexual people may believe that this option is not open to them. They see the heterosexual person being called on to delay sex, the homosexual person to forsake it. This can make the road more difficult for the homosexual person, but in those moments when sexual desire comes on most powerfully, I doubt if the struggles of homosexual and heterosexual individuals differ greatly. Furthermore, it is the homosexual identity, more than anything else, that leads the homosexual person to believe that fulfilling heterosexual marriage can never be open to him or her. In our ministry, most of the men, and many of the women, even in the early stages of their healing, believe that they will one day be married.

4. The prospect of change becomes less likely. Maybe I can change what I do, perhaps even change some of my feelings, but I cannot change who I am. Based on the number of people who come to ministries like Regeneration and to the hundred or so similar ministries in the United States and Canada, relative to the entire homosexual population, we have to believe that most homosexual people never consider change.

In one respect this is surprising. Especially for men, the homosexual life presents some horrible disadvantages. The extraordinary level of sexual promiscuity among homosexual men certainly indicates that they are never really meeting the needs that drive them. Homosexual men face terrible risks of disease and early death from their behavior, behavior that so many of them find themselves unable to stop. High rates of alcoholism, drug use, and suicide, much higher than among heterosexual people, all point to a life filled with emotional pain and stress. The focus on youth and beauty, the superficiality of much of the gay life, the powerful jealousies and dependencies (especially among women) all point to a life from which you would think people would want to escape – at least on their bad days.[4]

But relatively few seek a way out, either through our ministries or through secular therapies. I believe that there are several reasons for this, the most of important of which is that, for most homosexual people, the thought of being anyone else is unfathomable. I have discussed with homosexual people all of the evidence indicating that change is possible, I have shared my own story with them and pointed to others who have changed, I have explained some of the roots of homosexuality, and they may have identified with some of them, but at the end of the conversation they leave saying, "But it's who I am." So firm is that identity that they cannot even imagine it being otherwise.

Gay activists and their sympathizers actively promote the concept that change is impossible. The fact is, *every study attempting to measure the effectiveness of change therapies or religiously focused min - istries of change has revealed a significant success rate.*[5] Gays and their allies – some of them in the psychological and psychiatric fields – nevertheless keep claiming that change is impossible. No doubt, many of these individuals are motivated by a need to justify living the life that they themselves have chosen. With many such individuals, grasping the gay identity is a way to avoid having to face the hard questions that the possibility of change brings up.

5. It is living a lie. It is a lie because the gay identity is a false solution to real problems.

There are reasons why people grow up to have homosexual

attractions. Dr. Satinover and others believe that homosexuality is multi-causal, that is, a combination of factors contribute to homosexuality. The mixture of these factors differs from person to person, but we can identify certain factors that occur quite frequently. If there are genetic contributions in this mixture, they are probably secondary, and almost certainly they do not directly cause homosexuality. For example, a boy born with a passive personality, if he grows up in a certain family environment, might make decisions that would lead to homosexuality, while his more aggressive brother in the same environment would make different decisions. A girl who has an aggressive nature and exceptional athletic skills might be socialized by her family and friends into assuming manly roles, pushing her toward lesbianism.

The great majority of us who work in the field of helping people overcome homosexuality believe that the most influential factors leading to homosexuality are environmental or developmental. A girl, for example, is sexually molested as a child and grows up with a great fear and distrust of men. She comes to believe that her sexual and intimacy needs can only be met by another woman. A boy experiences real or perceived rejection by his father, or he does not gain affirmation from his father or from peers, and so he lives with an unmet need for a man's love or affirmation. Around the time of puberty this need becomes sexualized. A boy has a normal little boy's normal desire to be a man, but circumstances have convinced him that manhood can never be his, so he becomes driven to seek the manhood of other men.

My intention here is not to get into the causes of homosexuality – both Dr. Satinover and Dr. Nicolosi do this more than adequately earlier in this book – but to point out that within each homosexual person there are some problems that must be dealt with if that individual is to live a full, rich, and fulfilling life. Embracing a gay identity is a false answer to these problems. So many homosexual people spend their lives thinking that the next Mr. Right or the next strong woman will fill the huge empty place or heal the gaping wound that they have carried around for so many years. They have fallen for a lie, embracing homosexuality, when what they truly need is healing, forgiveness, the power to forgive others, the strength to venture out again into the real world of men and women, wholesome same-sex friendships, recognition of their true God-given manhood or womanhood, and above all, an intimate relationship with the Lord who loves and accepts them. Herein lie the true solutions to the real problems.

Once Established, Can One Escape from the Identity?

There are probably few things more difficult to change than a long established, deep-seated identity. Whether it is an identity as an American or as a Catholic, as a very fine person or as a miserable wretch, our identity dwells in the deep places that simple rational thinking or logic can seldom touch directly. My mother came to America as a young woman in 1919. She did not become a citizen until 1942. She married an American, was raising two American sons, and lived in America for more than twenty years, but it was only after the U.S. entered World War II that she knew it was "her country" that had entered the war; she became a U.S. citizen. It took her more than twenty years to change her national identity. How much more difficult it must be to change something else so much more central to our being – our sexual or gender identity.

One could say that our identity is a filter through which we view all of reality, but I believe that a pane of glass might offer a better analogy. We view life through the glass, but the glass itself is almost invisible; it just "is." Our identity just "is" but it gives us our reasons and justifications for what we do; gives rise to our affections and prejudices. If a homosexual man feels like a little boy inside, he will want some big strong man to hold him and protect him. If a woman carries the identity of a victim, she will structure her life around protecting herself from hurt. We may try to change our longings and feelings, but they are so difficult to change because they are a product of who we believe ourselves to be at the deepest level.

Many homosexual people can trace their homosexual feelings back to early childhood. Although at the time they did not translate these feeling into "being homosexual," retrospectively they do that. After they declare themselves gay, they look back and decide that they have always been this way. This powerfully reinforces the identity.

Further contributing to the solidification of a gay identity is the fact that we live in a culture that has exalted sexuality. Through the media, advertising, and other means of communication, our sexuality, rather than being a delightful gift to a man and woman who are married, becomes the central factor in life. If it is so important and central, shouldn't our sexuality then govern our identity?

So, when one's inner reality says that he is gay, and his environment increasingly supports this perspective, can a person who has once taken on a gay or lesbian identity let go of it and take on the identity of heterosexuality, or better yet, no longer define himself by his sexuality at all? Emphatically, I believe that he can. It has happened to me, and I have seen it happen to many, many others.

But it is a difficult process and usually a long one. To give up any identity is radical surgery, and if the identity brought such feelings of relief and joy when first taken on, change will, indeed, be difficult. It is not a five-step process; it is more of a whole life change, but let me describe five elements that will be a part of the process:

1. *Consciously dropping the identity.* One of the things we came to understand early on in ministries like Regeneration was that, if we were going to overcome homosexuality, we had to stop talking about ourselves that way. Although we have great respect for the Alcoholics Anonymous twelve steps – they are valid for overcoming any life-dominating condition – we always differed from AA and other traditional twelve-step programs in that we would never stand before one of our groups and say, "Hi, my name is Alan Medinger, and I am a homosexual." The identity is a part of the problem and letting it go, at least at the conscious level, is one of our first steps.

2. *Breaking certain ties.* One cannot continue to hang out at the gay bar, belong to the gay medical association, and play in the gay volleyball league and expect to see one's identity change. Those

associations that exist on the basis that the members or participants are all gay will have to be left behind, as painful as this may be. In our ministry, we seldom tell people that they have to give up their homosexual friends, but we find that, as a person's identity starts to change and he (or she) expands his world beyond the old gay environment, the only relationships with former homosexual friends that endure are those that were based on much more solid substance than a shared homosexuality.

3. *Coming to believe that being gay or lesbian is a false identity.* Serious, logical thought should bring a person to this conclusion, but as most honest people know, logic doesn't govern all of our decisions. Emotions are a big factor, as is our will – believing what we want to believe. Time and prayer may be needed to start to bring this truth into a person's heart. To try and help people in our ministry along in this process, a few years ago I wrote the following (which is about 70 percent true):

*   *   *   *   *   *   *   *   *   *   *   *   *   *

I Am Not an Accountant[6]

Ten years ago I left the business world to become full time Director of Regeneration.

I had been an accountant. I majored in accounting in college, passed the CPA exam a few years later. I worked as an accountant for one company for 4 years; then for a second for 22. Although I rose up into financial management, becoming controller, then treasurer and finally financial vice-president, I always had some involvement with accounting, and in my heart I was an accountant.

Most of my friends were accountants. Most days I ate lunch with other accountants. My wife's and my social life involved other accountants and their wives (later women accountants and their husbands – but that wasn't quite the same). We went to accounting dinners and dances. We went on trips sponsored by the accounting association.

I belonged to an accountant's Republican club, played in the accountant's volleyball league, and I was a coin col-lector, so I joined the accountant's coin collecting club. For a while as a young accountant I belonged to a political pres-sure group – the Accountants Defense League. This group had been formed to combat the prejudice and stereotyping aimed at accountants. We were constantly being pictured as pale, skinny, meek little Uriah Heep types, shoved off somewhere into the back room of an office, poring over our figures with a green eyeshade to protect us from the single bare bulb glaring down on our paper-strewn desks.

We protested whenever the media portrayed us this way. We declared that we were just like everybody else, and we publicized rugged athletes who had studied accounting, or hard hitting businessmen who had risen up from accounting to leadership in great corporations.

This was our public stance. We were like everybody else. But to be perfectly honest, we weren't fully convinced of this. We knew that we really were more comfortable around each other. Somehow we were different. When no one else was around at a gathering, sometimes we'd all put on our green eyeshades, relax and have a high old time. But 10 years ago, when entering full-time ministry, I left all that. I gave up that old identity. It wasn't easy – especially when I had to burn the green eyeshade. I kept some old accounting friends, but I resigned from the accounting association, the accountant's coin collecting club and all the rest. It shocked – even angered – my accountant friends. They felt I was turning my back on them. Vehemently, they tried to talk me out of what I was doing. "This is unnatu-ral," they declared. "You are denying who you really are. It will never work. You may repress your accountancy for a while, but you'll be miserable – or you'll be back."

It was difficult. How do you change who you perceive yourself to be? If I wasn't an accountant, who was I? At times I felt like I had no identity. I still felt so different from non-accountants. But gradually the change took place. As I became surrounded by other non-accountants who loved and accepted me as I was, and as God kept reminding me that accounting was what I did, not who I was, I gradual - ly started to change. That was 10 years ago, and truly, I no longer define myself as an accountant. It was what I did, not who I was. Sure, once in a while I would get the urge to jump in and balance a set of books, and I still believe I could complete a tax return with the best of them. But, that's not who I am.

Who am I? I am a husband, a father, a grandfather, a brother, a friend. I am a born-again, Spirit-filled believer in Jesus Christ. I am a member of the Body of Christ. I am a son of the King. I am one of the redeemed of the Lord. I am an American. I am Alan Medinger, and I am a creation of God, and I am unique in all the world. That's who I am. God has shown me that I am much more than I thought I was.

*   *   *   *   *   *   *   *   *   *   *   *   *   *   *

4. Focusing on who you are. Just as with the accountant, each of us is many more things than a homosexual – many of them far more indicative of who we truly are than our sexual orientation. Ponder these things. Every cell in a person's body marks him or her as male or female, as does the way we are put together, not just as regards our role in reproduction, but muscles, fat, brain struc- ture, countless ways.

In prayer we need to consider who God says we are. He creat- ed us male and female, both are good, both are made in His image. He equipped each gender with special gifts and He made men and women to have a wonderful complementarity. He longs to see His sons and daughters grow into the fullness of their manhood or womanhood. There is no place for homosexuality in this plan.

5. Living the life. Nature does abhor a vacuum. Vacuums have a tendency to cave in on themselves. The person who is giving up an old identity must take on, and learn to walk in, a new one.

What identity does a person take on when he or she abandons a homosexual identity? It is simple; the new identity is Man or Woman. We start to live as men and women in the world where we are placed. This does not mean blind conformity to some cultural stereotype – God loves our individuality – but it does mean that we learn to fulfill the obligations and legitimate expectations laid down for us as men and women. For our own good, for our own healing, we start to move in the world of healthy men and healthy women. Many of us found in this world – especially among fellow Christians – the affirmation that we so longed for and that is so necessary for our further healing.

What is suggested here is not a program of denial. Homosexual longings and attractions are real and can be enormously powerful. The opposite sex may offer absolutely no physical attractions to some people, but still this does not have to be the basis for making homosexuality an identity that governs the nature and scope of all our relationships.

Letting Go of the Identity by Parents and Loved Ones

At the beginning of this chapter I mentioned that the parent receiving the Thanksgiving or Christmas holiday news might, at first, want to assume that what they have heard is not real, or at worst is just a temporary phenomenon. Then coming to believe that the condition is more deeply rooted than they had hoped, the parents go through many of the stages of grieving; anger with God, anger with the child, guilt, bargaining with God, and so forth.

Some parents are overcome by the fact that they never suspected this about their child. They bounce back and forth between feeling that their child had betrayed them by his or her deception, and wondering at how they could have been so blind. "All of her life she never let me know who she was." "He was such a good boy, and now this." "I never knew my own child." Although these feelings are understandable, they are false. In fact the parents did know their child, they just didn't know this one thing about them: the direction of the child's sexual attractions. The sense of never having known the child means that the parents have absorbed the societal view that a person's homosexual feelings define the person. This is only one part of their child; it is not who he or she is.

When parents feel that they never really knew their child, it may be time to pull back and try to separate who their child is from his or her homosexuality.

I mentioned earlier that Christian parents who have just found out about a child's homosexuality are the most hurting people we minister to. Often central to this hurt is the question, "What did I do wrong?" Of course this parent, like every other parent did do some things wrong. The correct response to having done wrong, however, is not to embrace the child's gay identity, but confession and repentance. I don't believe there is a parent anywhere who wouldn't be eternally grateful for a second chance to do some things different with their children. I know that I would. All parents do make mistakes, but no parent *makes* a child turn out to be homosexual. But, telling parents this doesn't always bring relief from the guilt.

What does bring relief, or at least cover it up, however, is to believe that the child was born to be homosexual, that nothing could have changed this and that this is just the way he or she is. Gay is who he or she is, and it is unchangeable. Parents are often told this by well-meaning friends, often even by their clergy. This approach is the bread and butter of Parents and Friends of Lesbians and Gays (PFLAG). Attending a PFLAG meeting just after finding out about the child's homosexuality can bring great comfort to the heartbroken parents, but it is comfort based on a tragic misconception. By their beliefs, PFLAG people would sentence the people they love to a lifetime of homosexuality.

Besides, relieving parents of feelings of guilt, embracing their child's homosexuality brings comfort in several other ways. First, no parent wants to believe that his or her child is in serious sin and is leading a life in rebellion against God. How much better if this is the child's nature, and so the Church must be wrong.

Secondly, we live in a culture in which the only absolute virtue seems to be tolerance. The parents who embrace their child's homosexuality can feel good about how tolerant they are. I have seen the smug tolerance of "accepting" parents sitting in judgment of the narrow-minded parents who believe the Church's teaching on homosexuality. Finally, embracing the child's homosexuality avoids conflict and may win the approval of the child.

Brave and faithful are the parents who resist all of these temptations. Fortunately for them and for their child, the way of truth yields the better fruit in the long run.

I have seen parents pray their children out of homosexuality, but I have never seen them talk them out of it. By the same token, they cannot talk the child out of the identity once the child is an adult and has embraced it – unless the child is already wanting to leave homosexuality. So, what is the good fruit that can be borne by accepting the child, but not his or her homosexuality? It can come in several ways.

First, it helps the parents to see the child as a whole person instead of "the homosexual" child. It keeps homosexuality from crowding out everything else good and bad about the child, and it enables the parent to regard this child from the same perspective as they regard their other children.

Second, although parents may not be able to talk the child out of homosexuality, at least they will not be helping to solidify the identity. And the parents' demonstration that someone can love them and not accept their homosexual identity may provide one little chink in the armor that defends the child's false identity.

Finally, seeing homosexuality as sinful behavior and not as an identity may lead the parent to focus on what is most likely the greater problem in their child's life – the spiritual problem. In our ministry we always tell parents that if they have a child who is homosexual, but who does not have a real relationship with Christ, the number one issue is not homosexuality, it is Jesus Christ. The parents' first prayers need to be for the child to come back to the Church and to God. Only after this is the child likely to discover his or her true identity and want to live according to that identity.

Jesus tells us in *John* 8:32 that, "You shall know the truth, and the truth shall set you free." Taking on a gay or lesbian identity is a deception. It is not the truth. It clouds one's self-perception, and it can be a huge obstacle in a person's coming to know who he or she really is; a man or woman beloved by God and designed by Him for a special purpose – as a man or as a woman.

Endnotes

1. See, *Homosexuality and the Politics of Truth* (Grand Rapids: Baker Books, 1996), and also Chapter 1 of this book.

2. For a study on the occurrence and acceptance of homosexuality throughout history, see Greenberg, David F., *The Construction of Homosexuality*) Chicago: University of Chicago Press, 1988).

3. For a summary on recent data on promiscuity among homosexual men see: Schmidt, Thomas E., *Straight and Narrow?* (Downer's Grove: InterVarsity Press, 1995): 105–8.

4. For statistics on the occurrence of various pathologies associated with homosexuality (suicide, drug use, disease, etc.), see Maddoux, Marlin and Corbett, Christopher, *Answer to the Gay Deception* (International Christian Media, 1994) and Mazzalongo, Mike, Editor, *Gay Rights or Wrongs,* (College Press, 1995).

5. Goetze, Rob, *Homosexuality and the Possibility of Change: A Review of 17 Published Studies* on the internet, www.execulink.com/-newdirec/articles.hcm (Toronto: New Directions for Life, 1997–98) and subsequent addendum, *Another Six Studies* (1998).

6. "I Am Not an Accountant" *Regeneration News*, November 1994, (Baltimore, Regeneration). This monthy newsletter featuring articles offering help to people overcoming homosexuality is available at no charge by writing to Regeneration, P.O. Box 9830, Baltimore, MD 21284-9830; e-mail: regenbalto@juno.com.

Questions and Answers for Parents of Persons with Same-Sex Attractions
John F. Harvey, OSFS

From listening to parents with sons or daughters who have identified themselves as gay or lesbian, I have selected some frequently asked questions by such parents. I believe it will be helpful to respond to such questions, keeping in mind the differences between grown children and adolescent men and women.

1. What is homosexuality?

There are many definitions of homosexuality. "Traditionally, homosexuality has been described as a persistent and predominant attraction of a sexual-genital nature to persons of one's own sex. I use the term predominant to indicate that there may be a lesser degree of erotic interest in the other sex. . . . I use the term persistent to indicate that these erotic feelings toward someone of the same sex have persisted beyond the adolescent phase" (John F. Harvey, *The Homosexual Person*, San Francisco: Ignatius Press, 1987, p. 27).

Dr. Elizabeth Moberly, however, challenges the traditional understanding of homosexuality. She sees the condition of homosexuality as rooted in parent-child relationships, particularly in the early years of life. Moberly holds that the underlying factor in the development of same-sex relationships is that the person has suffered from some deficit in the relationship with the parental figure of the *same sex* and that there is a corresponding drive to make good this deficit through the medium of same-sex relationships (*Homosexuality: A New Christian Ethic*, Cambridge, England: James Clarke, 1983, p. 4).

2. Is homosexuality a sin?

One must carefully distinguish between the condition of homosexuality and homosexual acts. The condition of same-sex attraction is not a sin, but it is an objective disorder in the adolescent or adult person. If one gives in to the desire for same-sex acts one always sins. Homogenital acts are evil by their very nature. That is why the inclination to such acts, although *not* sinful, is an *objective disorder* (Sacred Congregation of the Doctrine of the Faith, *Letter to the Bishops of the Catholic Church on the Pastoral Care of Homosexual Persons*, 1986, sect. 3). Some persons attempt to dilute the meaning of objective disorder by saying that any sin of lust is an objective disorder; thus, if a man lusts for a woman, or vice versa, this is an objective disorder. Yes, it is a serious sin, but not a disorder, since the *inclination* of man for woman is good and natural when it is expressed in marriage.

The reason why homosexual acts are evil by their very nature is that they do not fulfill the two basic purposes of human sexual-genital acts, namely, the union of man and wife in marriage and the hope of children. One may say, then, that homogenital acts are seriously sinful. If, however, the individual involved in such acts is not aware of their malice, or has lost control of his will, he may not be guilty of mortal sin. Nevertheless he has the obligation to seek moral truth and to use the means of overcoming his compulsive tendencies.

3. Where is it stated in Church teaching that all homogenital acts are seriously and objectively sinful?

In the *Letter to the Romans,* Saint Paul describes various sins that blind the mind and lead to perverted activity. He includes homogenital acts by men and women (1, 18–27). The Sacred Congregation of the Doctrine of the Faith says that homogenital acts lack the indispensable finality of sexual activity, namely, the purpose of union between a man and a woman and the procreation of children ("Declaration on Certain Questions Concerning Sexual Ethics," 1975, sect. 8).

The same congregation developed this teaching in its 1986 letter, stressing that homogenital activity was "intrinsically" disordered, or always immoral by its very nature. As already pointed out, even the inclination to homogenital acts is an objective disorder, although the inclination itself is not sinful.

It should be noted, however, that persons who are involved in homogenital activity may not incur grave guilt, if they are unaware of the objective gravity of such acts, or if they are the slaves of compulsive tendencies which may handicap them for years. It is necessary that such persons seek help from group spiritual support systems like *Sexaholics Anonymous* and *Courage*.

4. Does not the culture regard sexual abstinence by anyone, heterosexual or homosexual, as virtually impossible?

To be sure, the culture looks suspiciously at anyone who claims to live a chaste life. A television hostess challenged a priest who advocated a life of sexual abstinence. When he responded with the assertion that he was happy living a celibate life, the hostess said that the priest was either neurotic or had a low sex drive. In short, the practice of sexual abstinence depends upon *motiva - tion*.

Persons of homosexual inclination should practice sexual abstinence out of love for Christ. If one makes a vow or promise to abstain from sexual activity because of love for Christ, then this person may be regarded as living a life of consecrated chastity or celibacy. There are many men and women doing just that.

5. But as a parent of a son or daughter with same-sex attractions I worry whether he will have an empty, lonely life if he tries to remain chaste. Actually everyone needs intimacy and companionship. Am I right?

You are correct. Everyone needs true friends and companions on the journey of life. But one can find friendship with other humans without the need for sexual-genital expression. To be sure, the sexual drive is strong, because for the majority of the human race it leads to marriage.

Many persons, moreover, with homosexual inclinations have to struggle to resist their desires for homosexual union. With the grace of God and group support and chaste friendships, members of Courage have found both peace and a measure of happiness – rooted in a personal prayer life.

6. What should parents do when their teenage son or daughter claims to be gay or lesbian?

In this situation Catholic parents should ask their child to seek spiritual direction and psychological guidance from priests and psychologists who are faithful to Church teaching. Parents have a right to exercise such authority in the face of objections by their child. It is a critical point in the child's life, although he may not agree with his parents' directive. This should *not be an option* for the child, but more a matter of obedience. The teenager is in no position to make a reliable evaluation of his own tendencies. Parents should inquire concerning the relationships of their child and the sources of information or misinformation that he is using. Oftentimes the teenager has browsed the Internet or covertly visited haunts, such as gay bars or homosexual movie theaters. Sometimes the teenager has been seduced by an older person, and is afraid to disclose this relationship to his parents.

7. Are we parents to blame for our son or daughter's homosexuality?

Many parents express their feelings of guilt to their counselor. They have heard that homosexual tendencies are inherited, or are the result of bad relationships with parents in early childhood. The honest answer is that in any given personal history there are many contributing factors: lack of same-sex peer relationships, lack of affection in the home, early seduction, traumatic experiences with strangers or with relatives, and so on. That is why, as a priest, I can tell a couple that we cannot say with certitude that John Jones is homosexual because he has never had a good relationship with his father. Very probably a number of factors, some of them *unknown* to the counselor, *converge* to bring about same-sex attraction in this individual. But only God really knows all the factors.

8. How did this happen to my child?

As explained above, professional therapists can make educated guesses concerning the origins of the homosexual condition.

About seventy-five years of research favors familial and environmental factors as the most important factors in the development of same-sex attraction.

9. Can homosexuality be prevented?

A recent book, *An Ounce of Prevention: Preventing the Homosexual Condition in Today's Youth* by Don Schmierer (Nashville: Word Publishing, 1998) collects works from a number of authors who have researched this question and have found that there are positive ways of preventing the development of same-sex attractions in the growing child.

Schmierer sees faulty family relationships as the source of same-sex attractions. He makes use of case histories to illustrate the ways in which adolescent boys and girls can have a confused perception of their gender identity. He shows how incest can push a teenaged daughter toward same-sex attractions because of her hatred of her father's behavior. He also describes certain situations which converge to indicate that a child is moving toward homosexuality; for example, a ten-year-old boy who is mocked by his peers for effeminate mannerisms. The same youngster is seen hanging out with girls exclusively. Effeminate behavior in boys is usually joined with a pattern of solitary behavior, i.e., the boy is known as a "loner" by his classmates.

The fatherless home or the emotionally unavailable father joined with the dominant mother contributes to the development of same-sex attractions in the male child and adolescent. Often where divorce has taken place, the mother portrays her ex-husband in very negative ways, and consequently the son loses respect for his father. I counseled a young lady (an only child whose father wanted a boy) who remembers her childhood as one in which she was constantly in the presence of boys in athletic contests. She did not associate with girls all through grade school. Later she found herself defending her mother against her alcoholic father, and on graduation from college she entered the lesbian lifestyle.

In merged or foster families one notices relationships among siblings, cousins, or neighbors that are compulsive and secretive and that can foster same-sex attractions. There are also young girls with much older female "best friends," while other girls of the same age are excluded. From these and other situations we gain insight concerning ways in which we can prevent or impede the growth of same-sex attractions in young men or women.

In the second part of his book Schmierer suggests ways in which we can create a loving home – a home where father and mother fulfill their responsibilities as parents, and where there are healthy communications among the children.

He encourages parents to be open and honest about personal struggles. True, this requires *discernment* and *wisdom*, but one's willingness to share personal concerns with children draws one closer to them. Let them know that their relationship with their parents is the most important element. Despite disagreements parents need to let their children know that they continue to love them.

In a chapter entitled "More Than Meets the Eye" Schmierer points out that "the list of possible influences that set the stage for a homosexual condition, Schmierer sums up these other influences:

A. *The individual person's self-will.* Sometimes the free will choices of children do not reflect the *values* of their parents, as does happen in this question of homosexuality.

B. *Verbal abuse by husband against wife or vice versa.* Damage can be done by either spouse against the other. Sometimes the mother abuses her husband in the presence of her son. The son may sympathize and identify with the mother's hurt – particularly if he has little attachment to the father. What follows, according to Dr. Nicolosi, is a mother and son united against the father. The boy will see masculinity as brutal and insensitive and be more inclined to reject his own manifestations of gender" (J. Nicolosi, *Reparative Therapy of Male Homosexuality*, 82–83).

C. *Sexual abuse and pedophilia.* Studies indicate that 50 percent of females have been molested before the age of twelve – most of them incestuously. In some studies it is pointed out that 58 percent or more of those in the homosexual lifestyle have been sexually abused in their developing years. Even if these figures are inflated, one may discern from life histories of abused individuals that pedophilic actions often lead to either *heterosexual* or *homosexual* promiscuity.

D. Other contributing factors include:

(1) *The infidelity of either parent*, especially as it impacts on the adolescent man or woman;

(2) *Moral relativism.* Beyond religious communities, there are no fixed standards or norms. Everything is relative. In *Generation Next* (Ventura: Regal Books, 1995) George Barna expresses the prevalent attitude toward truth: "Most Americans believe that all truth is relative to the situation and the individuals involved. Similarly, at least three quarters of our teens embrace the same position regarding moral truths. Not only do more than three out of four teenagers say there is no absolute moral truth; four out of five also claim nobody can know for certain whether or not they actually know what truth is . . ." (31; quoted by Schmierer, *op.cit.* 171–72). Barna notes that "Today's youth are likely to describe themselves as moral, not because of what they do, but because of how they *feel* . . . they live in accordance with situational ethics and moral relativism." (48; quoted by Schmierer, *op. cit.*, 172, italics added).

(3) *Peer pressure at the junior high and high school level.* "As young people seek for personal identity and acceptance, being liked is a powerful influence" (Schmierer, 173).

(4) *Temptation.* From his experience and observation Schmierer believes that one is most vulnerable to temptation after an emotional high. In *How Will I Tell My Mother?* Jerry Arterburn, who later died of AIDS, recounts a personal incident involving the aftermath of an emotional high.

(5) *Poor eye-to-hand coordination.* Men who are involved in the homosexual lifestyle often refer to early rejections on the playground as the beginning of their problems with gender identity. These men often lacked eye-to-hand coordination as children, and felt rejection by their peers deeply.

(6) *Chemical imbalances.* This is a very complex issue discussed by George Rekers in his *Handbook on Child and Adolescent Sexual*

Problems (New York: Lexington Books, 1995). The book addresses genetic, hormonal, and anatomic anomalies of the reproductive organs as well as the psychological effects related to these defects.

(7) *Failure of moral leadership.* This should include those moral leaders who have provided false information and destructive advice concerning the nature of same-sex attractions and homosexual acts.

Conclusion: Two authors have made landmark contributions concerning the origins and prevention of same-sex attractions, In *Psychogenesis: The Early Development of Gender Identity* (London: Routledge, 1983), Elizabeth Moberly suggests a series of ways in which same-sex attractions can be discovered in the very early years of the child (78–87). She stresses the need for a good gender relationship with the parent of the same sex.

George Rekers goes beyond the parental relationships to analyze the complexities of peer relationships as they impact on gender development. He is careful to avoid broad sweeping statements, because his many years of research have uncovered many different influences on the child and adolescent. He discusses not only the relationship of the child to the father, but also how the *child* sees the father-mother relationship. He centers his inquiry on gender-conformative, or non-conformative, behavior. This he finds has a *strong* association with the formation of same-sex attractions. Referencing the 1984 study, *Sexual Preference: Its Development in Men and Women* by Alan Bell, Martin Weinberg and Sue Hammersmith, Rekers tentatively concludes that "the main source for gender and sexual behavior deviance is found in social learning and psychological development variables . . . although we should recognize that there remains the theoretical possibility that biological abnormalities could contribute a potential vulnerability factor in some indirect way." (George Rekers, "The Formation of a Homosexual Orientation" in *Hope for Homosexuality* [Washington, D.C.: Free Congress Research, 1988], 18.)

10. Is "change" possible?
Generally, when parents ask this question, they are hoping their child will be able to get rid of the condition. But there is another

kind of change which can take place by the help of God's grace, and that is the development of the virtue of interior chastity, or purity of heart. This virtue is God's gift. It helps a person to avoid not only external acts of impurity, but also *deliberate* entertainment of lustful fantasies. As one grows in the love of Christ, one's thoughts and affections turn quickly to Christ in moments of temptation.

If "change" means moving out of same-sex attractions and developing heterosexual inclinations, then one should take a very qualified approach. This is a difficult kind of change. Among highly motivated individuals who seek to make this change through prayer, therapy and group support, it has been shown that one out of three persons was able to complete his or her psychosexual development into heterosexuality (1997 report of a two-year study by the National Association for Research and Therapy of Homosexuality; Joseph Nicolosi, Ph.D, Executive Director). But it is important to note that change of orientation is not a goal of Courage. We encourage individuals who seek to move away from homosexuality. But we do not make such change an obligation. It remains an option. The National Association of Research and Therapy of Homosexuality (NARTH) study also shows that another third show considerable improvement as a result of therapy.

11. My son in the gay lifestyle claims that he was born gay because ever since he can remember, he was attracted to other males. How do I respond to him?

It may be true that he has had same-sex attractions since he was very young. But that does not prove that he was born homosexual. For seventy-five years or more, volumes of research indicate that there are many environmental factors which contribute to the psychosexual formation of the person. I shall treat some of them later, but now I want to review briefly the research on genetic factors as described by Father Jeffrey Keefe, O.F.M. Conv., in chapter three of my book, *The Truth about Homosexuality* (San Francisco: Ignatius Press, 1996), pp. 31–67.

Father Keefe shows that none of the more recent research projects on the origins of homosexuality have discovered the homosexual gene, or cluster of genes. In *Homosexuality and the Politics of Truth* (Grand Rapids: Baker Books, 1996) Dr. Jeffrey Satinover says that we have little data indicating that homosexuality is due to a gene or even a cluster of genes.

Dr. Satinover rehearses his findings in Chapter 1 of this book.

12. In the case of someone who mentioned to his parish priest the feeling that he was "gay," the priest said some people are born this way. Is this really so?

As Father Jeffrey Keefe shows, there is no scientific evidence that one is born homosexual. In more recent years the popular press has published articles indicating that certain brain structures were linked to the condition of homosexuality. Studies of identical twins seemed to indicate a greater incidence of homosexuality among such twins until critics pointed out that the data submitted could be used just as well to indicate that their homosexual condition was formed by environmental factors.

13. Do environmental and familial factors contribute to the formation of same-sex attractions in men and women? Please elaborate.

Research and clinical psychologists are careful not to ascribe same-sex attractions to one single cause; they tend to see this condition as the result of a convergence of several factors within the psychosexual development of the individual.

Let me give you an example. George was the youngest son among five children, having three older brothers who were five, seven, and ten years older than he. He had a sister two years older. The father was a sports enthusiast who had coached the three older brothers in Little League baseball, but he was disappointed in George, who showed no interest in teamwork. In grade school George discerned that he was an awful baseball player, and gradually moved away from sports into the Internet. Again there was very little conversation between George and his father, who worked two jobs to put his children through Catholic schools.

George got into the Internet at twelve years old, not seeming to care that he was not with his male peers in rough house play or sports.

George moreover felt inferior to his older brothers and to his peers with whom he had no close association. His mother was concerned that he spent so much time in his room watching TV and on the Internet. As he moved into adolescence, he felt even more isolated from his male schoolmates who were always talking about girls. He felt that he was not like them. He wanted to be close to certain guys to whom he was physically attracted. But he was afraid to approach them.

The above account of a young man with same-sex attractions is classical. You may have noted that he yearned for male companionship, and that he had never identified with his father. These were contributing factors, but there were others, including his feelings of inferiority as masculine.

How these factors converge to form a homosexual orientation in this person is not clear. It is very probable that the factors that contributed to same-sex attractions in George are all psychological.

14. What kind of support is most beneficial for someone who has been actively engaged in homosexual acting out?

The best kind of support is found in Courage, which proposes a serious program for the development of the means of living chastely. The program places special emphasis on prayer of the heart every day, on regular meetings in which the members of the group speak about their own experiences and efforts to correspond with God's grace, and on the value of chaste friendships to preserve the life of interior prayer.

15. What can we do to help our grown child?

On the strictly human level it may seem that you can do very little to change the thinking of your *grown* son or daughter. Usually adult children have been in the lifestyle for some time before they inform their parents that they are gay or lesbian. It is best then to inform your grown child that you love him (her), but you do not accept homogenital behavior because it is seriously immoral. Convey that you hope your son or daughter is willing to reconsider acceptance of a lifestyle which cannot lead to lasting happiness in this world or the next. One should not hesitate to describe lasting happiness in terms of personal redemption in Christ. Parents should continue to keep in touch with the grown son or daughter without overdoing it by complaining that their child does not answer letters or return phone calls. Above all, parents should pray daily for their child.

16. What can priests do to help parents of grown sons or daughters who are in the lifestyle, i.e., in some kind of homogenital relationship?

The first thing a priest should do is to listen to the parents' story. Generally, the grown son or daughter has been in the lifestyle for some time before he or she reveals the situation to the parents. Oftentimes siblings already know. Sometimes the mother knows before the father. In any case it will be necessary for the priest to encourage the parents not to give up on their grown child, and also not to cave in to the demands of their offspring. Very probably the parents have been requested to accept their offspring's partner, and the parents have refused to do so, but are uncertain *how* to relate to their son or daughter.

The priest should advise the parents to keep in touch with their offspring, while doing nothing to approve the partnership. This is a delicate balance which their child may reject, because such a one wants complete approval of his sexual union. Generally, the parents express their love for their child, but continue to reject his sexual behavior.

17. Our son is living with another man. Both of them have discussed their relationship with a priest and a clinical psychologist. Each counseled that it is better to live with one person in a faithful relationship than to be involved in promiscuous one-night stands. What response do we give our son?

The priest and psychologist both assume that it is practically impossible for an adult with same-sex attractions to live a life of sexual abstinence. One moralist comments that such persons are entitled to some form of sexual intimacy, because they are *not* called to the life of consecrated celibacy, a calling given only to a few.

This solution, however, is contrary to authentic Catholic teaching in several ways. It ignores the divine command that each of us practice the virtue of chastity according to our state of life. Only in marriage may man and woman have sexual-genital intercourse. All other friendships are meant to be sexually abstinent, or celibate. To the objection that such is practically impossible, one must consider that God never imposes an obligation without giving the individual the grace to carry it out, St. Augustine expressed this truth in his *Confessions*: "Lord, give me the grace to do what you command, and command whatever you will" (Book X, Chapter 29). This teaching was reaffirmed in the Council of Trent (See *The Homosexual Person*, p. 83, n. 12 ; *The Truth about Homosexuality*, p. 198).

The lesser of two evils argument used by the priest and psychologist is erroneous. One may not apply this argument when we are dealing with an act which is evil by its very nature, as all homogenital acts are. The assumption, moreover, that such steady lover relationships will be exclusively faithful is contrary to the collective experience of male homosexual couples. Studies of such couples show that after the first five years of living together the couple began to be unfaithful to one another. The requirement of strict fidelity is dropped in favor of emotional bonding.

Again, why should we make exceptions for persons with same-sex attractions when it comes to the obligation of chastity? We do not make exception for many heterosexual men and women who, for serious reasons of family circumstances or health, physical and mental, do not practice the virtue of chastity. All are bound to chastity, and God will give them the grace to fulfill His commandment.

18. Our daughter, 35, is in a same-sex partnership for the last three years. Though we parents do not approve of our daughter's same-sex union, we make it clear that we love her, and we want to keep in contact with her. She, however, wants us to accept her lover into our home on a regular basis, and she wants us to visit them regularly as we do our married son's family.

The moral difficulty with parents and lesbian couples visiting one another regularly is that it creates the impression that the parents *approve* the lifestyle of their daughter. It is exactly what Parents and Friends of Gays and Lesbians (PFLAG) advocate, because PFLAG believes that parents ought to approve a gay or lesbian couple as normal and good.

As Catholics, parents should take reasonable steps to avoid *regular* visits to the home of such a couple. Their daughter may visit them as often as she desires, but *alone* as their daughter. On exceptional occasions, however, the daughter may bring her partner, but they should not be permitted to say overnight in the same bedroom. "Exceptional occasions" would seem to include Christmas visits, family reunions, and the like. It would be clear to the siblings in the family that this was *not* an approval of their sibling's lifestyle.

Some parents, however, would not allow even an exceptional visit, and they have a right to make this decision; nevertheless, as long as scandal is avoided, exceptional visits may be morally permitted.

No doubt, these are very sensitive issues, and all concerned should realize that both parents and the child with same-sex attractions are coming from very different philosophies of life. The parents' decision, however, is firmly rooted in their Faith.

19. What help does the Church provide for parents in the situation discussed in Question 18?

For the last ten years I have listened to parents in similar situations. In most instances the relationship between the adult child and the parents is at a stalemate. The adult child goes his own way, usually putting distance between himself and his parents and often rejecting his Catholic Faith as well. At this point parents need spiritual support, and that is why *EnCourage* was founded. It has given parents of grown sons and daughters a place to meet and to share with one another. The spiritual guidance of a priest-counselor is appreciated at these monthly meetings. Further information about *EnCourage*, including a list of contacts, may be obtained from the *Courage* office in New York, telephone 212-268-1010.

20. Where may parents find some good reading on homosexuality in its various aspects?

I select the following titles as *representative* of the many good books in the field; they are *not* listed alphabetically.

1. Jerry Arterburn, *How Will I Tell My Mother?* (Nashville: Thomas Nelson, 1988).
2. Barbara Johnson, *Where Does a Mother Go to Resign?* (Minneapolis: Bethany House Publishers, revised 1994).
3. Barbara Johnson, *Stick a Geranium in Your Hat and Be Happy.* (Nashville: Word Books, 1990).

(Both Johnson books are "must read" books.)

4. Leanne Payne, *Crisis in Masculinity* (Wheaton, Ill.: Crossway Books, 1985; reprinted Grand Rapids, Michigan: Baker Book House, 1996).
5. Leanne Payne, *The Broken Image: Restoring Personal Wholeness Through Healing Prayer* (1981: reprinted Grand Rapids, Mich.: Baker Book House, 1996).

   Superb treatment.

6. George Rekers, *Handbook of Child and Adolescent Sexual Problems* (New York: Lexington Books, 1995).
7. George Rekers, *The Formation of a Homosexual Orientation* (New York: Lexington Books, 1995).
8. Gerard van den Aardweg, *The Battle for Normality* (San Francisco: Ignatius Press, 1997).
9. Joseph Nicolosi, *Reparative Therapy of Male Homosexuality* (Northvale, N.J.: Jason Aronson, 1991; reprinted 1998).
10. Elizabeth Moberly, Homosexuality: A New Christian Ethic (Cambridge University Press, 1983; reprinted Greenwood, South Carolina: Attic Press, 1997).
11. John F. Harvey, OSFS, *The Homosexual Person* (San Francisco: Ignatius Press, 1987).
12. John Harvey, *The Truth about Homosexuality* (San Francisco: Ignatius Press, 1996).
13. Ed Hurst, *Homosexuality: Laying the Axe to the Roots* (privately published).
14. Jeff Konrad, *You Don't Have to Be Gay: Hope and Freedom for Males Struggling with Homosexuality or for Those Who Know of*

Someone Who Is (Newport Beach, CA: Pacific Publishing, 1987; revised 1992).

15. Joe Dallas, Desires in Conflict (Eugene, Ore.: Harvest House Publishers, 1991).

16. Joe Dallas, *A Strong Delusion* (Eugene, Ore.: Harvest House Publishers, 1996).

17. Bob Davies and Lori Rentzel, *Coming Out of Homosexuality* (Downer's Grove, Ill.: InterVarsity Press, 1993).

18. Jeanette Howard, *Out of Egypt: Leaving Lesbianism Behind* (Tunbridge Wells, Kent, United Kingdom: Monarch Publications, 1991; reprinted by Regeneration Books). The first ex-gay book to specifically treat lesbianism.

19. Lori Rentzel, *Emotional Dependency* (Downers Grove, Ill.: InterVarsity Press, 1990).

20. Briar Whitehead, *Craving for Love* (Tunbridge Wells, Kent, United Kingdom: Monarch Publications, 1993).

21. Don Schmierer, *An Ounce of Prevention: Preventing the Homosexual Condition in Today's Youth* (Nashville: Word Publishing Company, 1998).

22. Jeffrey Satinover, *Homosexuality and the Politics of Truth* (Grand Rapids: Baker Books, 1996).

23. Thomas Schmidt, *Straight and Narrow* (Downers Grove, Ill.: InterVarsity Press, 1995).

21. What are some positive suggestions for parents of persons with same-sex attractions?

First, don't panic when you learn that your child, whether youth or adult, claims to be gay or lesbian. You may have strong feelings of anger and fear, but be careful not to express them immediately to your child. Instead express love for your child. Bill Devlin, a Philadelphia minister, was debating a gay activist at a college campus when a young lady asked him what he would do if his oldest daughter came home and told him that she was in love with a woman. The minister replied that he would take her in his arms, tell her that he loved her – and always would – but that she had made a mistake and must break off the relationship. "There was a pause before the gay activist he was debating reduced the room to stunned silence by quietly beginning his response: 'I wish that Bill Devlin had been my father.'" (David Boldt, "Lovingly Fighting Gay Rights," *Philadelphia Inquirer*, October 30, 1998).

It is probable, however, that your child will want to talk about your disapproval of her lifestyle. She may be convinced that she has a right to a same-sex union. Then as a parent you calmly state your belief that all homogenital acts are seriously immoral. Try not to shout or scream, although your son or daughter may do so. After the conversation continue to show affection for your child. Give the child the opportunity to discuss the matter in the future. Pray always.

Second, seek information about *EnCourage* by calling the New York office at 212-268-1010, or write Courage, c/o St. John the Baptist Rectory, 210 West 31st Street, New York, NY 10001. Perhaps you may help form a unit of *EnCourage* in your locality. If possible, come to the Annual *Courage/EnCourage* Conference every August. Seek spiritual guidance from a priest who supports *Courage*. Check out the reading listed in Question 20, making sure you get Barbara Johnson's *Where Does a Mother Go to Resign?* and Don Schmierer's *An Ounce of Prevention*. Third, in communicating with your child with same-sex attractions do not sermonize or send loads of Courage materials. Remember him on his birthday, and during the Christmas season.

Appendices

Always Our Children
(Revised)

The purpose of this pastoral message is to reach out to parents who are trying to cope with the discovery of homosexuality in a child who is an adolescent or an adult. It urges families to draw upon the reservoirs of faith, hope, and love as they face uncharted futures. It asks them to recognize that the Church offers enormous spiritual resources to strengthen and support them at this moment in their family's life and in the days to come.

This message draws upon the *Catechism of the Catholic Church*, the teaching of Pope John Paul II, statements of the Congregation for the Doctrine of the Faith and of our own episcopal conference. The message is not a treatise on homosexuality. It is not a systematic presentation of the Church's moral teaching. It does not break any new ground theologically. Rather, relying on the Church's teaching as well as on our own pastoral experience, we intend to speak words of faith, hope, and love to parents who need the Church's loving presence at a time which may be one of the most challenging in their lives.

We also want to be helpful to priests and pastoral ministers, who often are the first ones parents or their children approach with their struggles and anxieties.

In recent years we have tried to reach out to families in difficult circumstances. Our initiatives took the form of short statements like this one, which were addressed to people who thought they were beyond the Church's circle of care. "Always Our Children" follows in the same tradition as these other pastoral statements.

This message is not intended for advocacy purposes or to serve a particular agenda. It is not to be understood as an endorsement of what some call a "homosexual lifestyle."

"Always Our Children" is an outstretched hand of the bishops' Committee on Marriage and Family to parents and other family members, offering them a fresh look at the grace present in family life and the unfailing mercy of Christ our Lord.

> "An even more generous, intelligent and prudent pastoral commitment modeled on the Good Shepherd is called for in cases of families which, often independent of their own wishes and through pressures of various other kinds, find themselves faced by situations which are objectively difficult" – Pope John Paul II, "On the Family," 77.

A Critical Moment, a Time of Grace

As you begin to read this message you may feel your life is in turmoil. You and your family might be faced with one of the difficult situations of which our Holy Father speaks:

–You think your adolescent child is experiencing a same-sex attraction and/or you observe attitudes and behaviors that you find confusing or upsetting or with which you disagree.

–Your son or daughter has made it known that he or she has a homosexual orientation.

–You experience a tension between loving your child as God's precious creation and not wanting to endorse any behavior you know the Church teaches is wrong.

You need not face his painful time alone without human assistance or God's grace. The Church can be an instrument of both help and healing. This is why we bishops, as pastors and teachers, write to you.

In this pastoral message we draw upon the gift of faith as well as the sound teaching and pastoral practice of the Church in order to offer loving support, reliable guidance and recommendations for ministries suited to your needs and those of your child. Our message speaks of accepting yourself, your beliefs and values, your questions, and all you may be struggling with at the moment; of accepting and loving your child as a gift of God; and of accepting the full truth of God's revelation about the dignity of the human person and the meaning of human sexuality. Within the Catholic moral visions there is no contradiction among these levels of acceptance, for truth and love are not opposed. They are inseparably joined and rooted in one person, Jesus Christ, who reveals God to be Ultimate Truth and Saving Love.

We address our message also to the wider Church community and especially to priests and other pastoral ministers, asking that our words be translated into attitudes and actions which follow the way of love as Christ has taught. It is through the community of his faithful that Jesus offers you hope, help, and healing so that your whole family might continue to grow into the intimate community of life and love which God intends.

Accepting Yourself

Because some of you might be swept up in a tide of emotions, we focus first on feelings. Although the gift of human sexuality can be a great mystery at times, the Church's teaching on homosexuality is clear. However, because the terms of that teaching have now become very personal in regard to your son or daughter, you may feel confused and conflicted.

Possibly you are experiencing many different emotions, all in varying degrees such as:

Relief: Perhaps you had sensed for some time that your son or daughter was different in some way. Now he or she has come to you and has entrusted something very significant. It may be that other siblings learned of this before you did and were reluctant to tell you. Regardless, though, a burden has been lifted. Acknowledge the possibility that your child has told you this not to hurt you or create distance, but out of love and trust and with a desire for honesty, intimacy, and closer communication.

Anger: You may be feeling deceived or manipulated by your son or daughter. You could be angry with your spouse, blaming him or her for "making the child this way"– especially if there has been a difficult parent-child relationship. You might be angry with yourself for not recognizing indications of homosexuality. You could be feeling disappointment, along with anger, if family members and sometimes even siblings are rejecting their homosexual brother or sister. It is just as possible to feel angry if family members or friends seem overly accepting and encouraging of homosexuality. Also – and not to be discounted – is a possible anger with God that all this is happening.

Mourning: You may now feel that your child is not exactly the same individual you once thought you knew. You envision that your son or daughter may never give you grandchildren. These lost expectations as well as the fact that homosexual persons often encounter discrimination and open hostility can cause you great sadness.

Fear: You may fear for your child's physical safety and general welfare in the face of prejudice against homosexual people. In particular, you may be afraid that others in your community might exclude or treat your child or your family with contempt. The fear of your child contracting HIV/AIDS or another sexually transmitted disease is serious and ever present. If your child is distraught, you may be concerned about attempted suicide.

Guilt, shame, and loneliness: "If only we had . . . or had not" are words with which parents can torture themselves at this time. Regrets and disappointments rise up like ghosts from the past. A sense of failure can lead you into a valley of shame which, in turn, can isolate you from your children, your family, and other communities of support.

Parental protectiveness and pride: Homosexual persons often experience discrimination and acts of violence in our society. As a parent, you naturally want to shield your children from harm, regardless of their age. You may still insist: "You are always my child; nothing can ever change that. You are also a child of God, gifted and called for a purpose in God's design."

There are two important things to keep in mind as you try to sort out your feelings. First, listen to them. They can contain clues leading to a fuller discovery of God's will for you. Second, because some feelings can be confusing or conflicting, it is not necessary to

212

act upon all of them. Acknowledging them may be sufficient, but it may also be necessary to talk about your feelings. Do not expect that all tensions can or will be resolved. The Christian life is a journey marked by perseverance and prayer. It is a path leading from where we are to where we know God is calling us.

Accepting Your Child

How can you best express your love – itself a reflection of God's unconditional love – for your child? At least two things are necessary.

First, don't break off contact; don't reject your child. A shocking number of homosexual youth end up on the streets because of rejection by their families. This and other external pressures can place young people at greater risk of self-destructive behaviors like substance abuse and suicide.

Your child may need you and the family now more than ever. He or she is still the same person. This child, who has always been God's gift to you, may now be the cause of another gift: your family becoming more honest, respectful, and supportive. Yes, your love can be tested by this reality, but it can also grow stronger through your struggle to respond lovingly.

The second way to communicate love is to seek appropriate help for your child and for yourself. If your son or daughter is an adolescent, it is possible that he or she may be displaying traits which cause you anxiety, such as what the child is choosing to read or view in the media, intense friendships, and other such observable characteristics and tendencies. What is called for on the part of parents is an approach which does not presume that your child has developed a homosexual orientation and which will help you maintain a loving relationship while you provide support, information, encouragement, and moral guidance. Parents must always be vigilant about their children's behavior and exercise responsible interventions when necessary.

In many cases it may be appropriate and necessary that your child receive professional help, including counseling, and spiritual direction. It is important, of course, that he or she receive such guidance willingly. Look for a therapist who has an appreciation of religious values and who understands the complex nature of sexuality. Such a person should be experienced at helping people discern the meaning of early sexual behaviors, sexual attractions, and sexual fantasies in ways that lead to more clarity and self-identity. In the course of this, however, it is essential for you to remain open to the possibility that your son or daughter is struggling to understand and accept a basic homosexual orientation.

The meaning and implications of the term *homosexual orientation* are not universally agreed upon. Church teaching acknowledges a distinction between a homosexual "tendency" which proves to be "transitory" and "homosexuals who are definitively such because of some kind of innate instinct" (Congregation for the Doctrine of the Faith, *Declaration on Certain Questions Concerning Sexual Ethics*, 8).

In light of this possibility, therefore, it seems appropriate to understand sexual orientation (heterosexual or homosexual) as a *deep-seated* dimension of one's personality and to recognize its relative stability in a person. A homosexual orientation produces a stronger emotional and sexual attraction toward individuals of the same sex rather than toward those of the opposite sex. It does not totally rule out interest in, care for, and attraction toward members of the opposite sex. Having a homosexual orientation does not necessarily mean a person will engage in homosexual activity.

There seems to be no single cause of a homosexual orientation. A common opinion of experts is that there are multiple factors – genetic, hormonal, psychological – that may give rise to it. Generally, homosexual orientation is experienced as a given, not as something freely chosen. By itself, therefore, a homosexual orientation cannot be considered sinful, for morality presumes the freedom to choose.

Some homosexual persons want to be known publicly as *gay* or *lesbian*. These terms often express a person's level of self-awareness and self-acceptance within society. Though you might find the terms offensive because of political or social connotations, it is necessary to be sensitive to how your son or daughter is using them. Language should not be a barrier to building trust and honest communication.

You can help a homosexual person in two general ways. First, encourage him or her to cooperate with God's grace in order to live a chaste life. Second, concentrate on the person, not on the homosexual orientation itself. This implies respecting a person's freedom to choose or refuse therapy directed toward changing a homosexual orientation. Given the present state of medical and psychological knowledge, there is no guarantee that such therapy will succeed. Thus, there may be no obligation to undertake it, though some may find it helpful.

All in all, it is essential to recall one basic truth. God loves every person as a unique individual. Sexual identity helps to define the unique persons we are. One component of our sexual identity is sexual orientation. Thus, our total personhood is more encompassing than sexual orientation. Human beings see the appearance, but the Lord looks into the heart (cf. 1 *Sm*, 16:7).

God does not love someone any less simply because he or she is homosexual. God's love is always and everywhere offered to those who are open to receiving it. St. Paul's words offer great hope:

> For I am convinced that neither death nor life, nor angels, nor principalities, nor present things, nor future things, nor powers, nor height, nor depth, nor any other creature will be able to separate us from the love of God in Christ Jesus our Lord (*Rom.* 8:38–9).

Accepting God's Plan and the Church's Ministry

For the Christian believer, an acceptance of self and of one's homosexual child must take place within the larger context of accepting divinely revealed truth about the dignity and destiny of human persons. It is the Church's responsibility to believe and teach this truth, presenting it as a comprehensive moral vision and applying this vision in particular situations through its pastoral ministries. We present the main points of that moral teaching here.

Every person has an inherent dignity because he or she is created in God's image. A deep respect for the total person leads the Church to hold and teach that sexuality is a gift of God. Being created a male or a female person is an essential part of the divine plan, for it is their sexuality – a mysterious blend of spirit and body – that allows human beings to share in God's own creative love and life.

Like all gifts from God, the power and freedom of sexuality can be channeled toward good or evil. Everyone – the homosexual and the heterosexual person – is called to personal maturity and responsibility. With the help of God's grace, everyone is called to practice the virtue of chastity in relationships. Chastity means integrating one's thoughts, feelings and actions in the area of human sexuality in a way that values and respects one's own dignity and that of others. It is "the spiritual power which frees love from selfishness and aggression" (Pontifical Council for the Family, "The Truth and Meaning of Human Sexuality," 16).

Christ summons all his followers – whether they are married or liv - ing a single celibate life – to a higher standard of loving. This includes not only fidelity, forgiveness, hope, perseverance, and sacrifice, but also chastity, which is expressed in modesty and self-control. The chaste life is possible, though not always easy, for it involves a continual effort to turn toward God and away from sin, especially with the strength of the Sacraments of Penance and Eucharist. Indeed God expects everyone to strive for the perfection of love, but to achieve it gradually through stages of moral growth (cf. John Paul II, "On the Family," 34). To keep our feet on the path of conversion, God's grace is available to and sufficient for everyone open to receiving it.

Furthermore, as homosexual persons "dedicate their lives to understanding the nature of God's personal call to them, they will be able to celebrate the sacrament of penance more faithfully and receive the Lord's grace so freely offered there in order to convert their lives more fully to his way" (Congregation for the Doctrine of the Faith, "The Pastoral Care of Homosexual Persons," 12).

To live and love chastely is to understand that "only within marriage does sexual intercourse fully symbolize the Creator's dual design as an act of covenant love with the potential of co-cre-ating new human life" (U.S. Catholic Conference, *Human Sexuality: A Catholic Perspective for Education and Lifelong Learning,* p. 55). This is a fundamental teaching of our Church about sexual-ity, rooted in the biblical account of man and woman created in the image of God and made for union with one another (*Gn.* 2–3).

Two conclusions follow. First, it is God's plan that sexual inter-course occur only within marriage between a man and a woman. Second, every act of intercourse must be open to the possible cre-ation of new human life. Homosexual intercourse cannot fulfill these two conditions. Therefore, the Church teaches that homogential behavior is objectively immoral, while making the important distinction between this behavior and a homosexual orientation, which is not immoral in itself.

It is also important to recognize that neither a homosexual ori-entation nor a heterosexual one leads inevitably to sexual activity. One's total personhood is not reducible to sexual orientation or behavior.

Respect for the God-given dignity of all persons means the recogni - tion of human rights and responsibilities. The teaching of the Church makes it clear that the fundamental human rights of homosexual persons must be defended and that all of us must strive to elimi-nate any form of injustice, oppression, or violence again them (cf. Congregation of the Doctrine of the Faith, "The Pastoral Care of Homosexual Persons," 10).

It is not sufficient only to avoid unjust discrimination. Homosexual persons "must be accepted with respect, compassion and sensitivity" (*Catechism of the Catholic Church,* 2358).

They, as is true of every human being, need to be nourished at many different levels simultaneously.

This includes friendship, which is a way of loving and is essential to healthy human development as well as one of the rich-est possible human experiences. Friendship can and does thrive outside of genital sexual involvement.

The Christian community should offer its homosexual sisters and brothers understanding and pastoral care. More than twenty years ago we bishops stated that "homosexuals . . . should have an active role in the Christian community" (National Conference of Catholic Bishops, "To Live in Christ Jesus: A Pastoral Reflection on the Moral Life," p. 19). What does this mean in practice? It means that all homosexual persons have a right to be welcomed into the community, to hear the word of God, and to receive pastoral care. Homosexual persons who are living chaste lives should have opportunities to lead and serve the community. However, the Church has the right to deny public roles of service and leadership to persons, whether homosexual or heterosexual, whose public behavior openly violates its teachings.

The Church recognizes the importance and urgency of ministering to persons with HIV/AIDS. Though HIV/AIDS is an epidemic affecting the whole human race, not just homosexual persons, it has had a devastating effect upon them and has brought great sorrow to many parents, families, and friends.

Without condoning self-destructive behavior or denying personal responsibility, we reject the idea that HIV/AIDS is a direct punishment from God. Furthermore: "Persons with AIDS are not distant, unfamiliar people, the objects of our mingled pity and aversion. We must keep them present to our consciousness as individuals and a community, and embrace them with unconditional love. . . . Compassion – love – toward persons infected with HIV is the only authentic Gospel response: (NCCB, "Called to Compassion and Responsibility: A Response to the HIV/AIDS Crisis").

Nothing in the Bible or in Catholic teaching can be used to justify prejudicial or discriminatory attitudes and behaviors. We reiterate here what we said in an earlier statement:

"We call on all Christians and citizens of good will to confront their own fears about homosexuality and to curb the humor and discrimination that offend homosexual persons. We understand that having a homosexual orientation brings with it enough anxiety, pain and issues related to self-acceptance without society bringing additional prejudicial treatment" (*Human Sexuality: A Catholic Perspective for Education and Lifelong Learning*, p. 55).

Pastoral Recommendations

With a view toward overcoming the isolation that you or your son or daughter may be experiencing, we offer these recommendations to you as well as to priests and pastoral ministers.

To parents:

1. Accept and love yourselves as parents in order to accept and love your son or daughter. Do not blame yourselves for a homosexual orientation in your child.

2. Do everything possible to continue demonstrating love for your child. However, accepting his or her homosexual orientation does not have to include approving all related attitudes and behavioral choices. In fact, you may need to challenge certain aspects of a lifestyle that you find objectionable.

3. Urge your son or daughter to stay joined to the Catholic faith community. If they have left the Church, urge them to return and be reconciled to the community, especially in the Sacrament of Penance.

4. Recommend that your son or daughter find a spiritual director/mentor who will offer guidance in prayer and in leading a chaste and virtuous life.

5. Seek help for yourself, perhaps in the form of counseling or spiritual direction, as you strive for understanding, acceptance and inner peace. Also, consider joining a parents' support group or participating in a retreat designed for Catholic parents of homosexual children. Other people have traveled the same road as you but may have journeyed even further. They can share effective ways of handling delicate family situations such as how to tell family members and friends about your child, how to explain homosexuality to younger children, and how to relate to your son or daughter's friends in a Christian way.

6. Reach out in love and service to other parents who may be struggling with a son's or daughter's homosexuality. Contact your parish about organizing a parents' support group. Your diocesan family ministry office, Catholic Charities, or a special diocesan ministry to gay and lesbian persons may be able to offer assistance.

7. As you take advantage of opportunities for education and support, remember that you can only change yourself; you can only be responsible for your own beliefs and actions, not those of your adult children.

8. Put your faith completely in God, who is more powerful, more compassionate, and more forgiving than we are or ever could be.

To Church ministers:

1. Be available to parents and families who ask for your pastoral help, spiritual guidance, and prayer.

2. Welcome homosexual persons into the faith community. Seek out those on the margins. Avoid stereotyping and condemnations. Strive first to listen. Do not presume that all homosexual persons are sexually active.

3. Learn about homosexuality and Church teaching so that your preaching, teaching, and counseling will be informed and effective.

4. When speaking publicly, use the words *homosexual, gay,* and *lesbian* in honest and accurate ways.

5. Maintain a list of agencies, community groups, and counselors or other experts to whom you can refer homosexual persons or their parents and family members when they ask you for specialized assistance.

6. Help to establish or promote existing support groups for parents and family members.

7. Learn about HIV/AIDS so you will be more informed and compassionate in your ministry. Include prayers in the liturgy for those living with HIV/AIDS, their caregivers, those who have died, and their families, companions, and friends. A special Mass for healing and anointing of the sick might be connected with World AIDS Awareness Day (December 1) or with a local AIDS-awareness program.

Conclusion

For St. Paul, love is the greatest of spiritual gifts. St. John considers love to be the most certain sign of God's presence. Jesus proposes it as the basis of his two great Commandments which fulfill all the law and the prophets.

Love, too, is the continuing story of every family's life. Love can be shared, nurtured, rejected, and sometimes lost. To follow Christ's way of love is the challenge before every family today. You family now has an added opportunity to share love and to accept love. Our Church communities are likewise called to an exemplary standard of love and justice. Our homosexual sisters and brothers – indeed, all people – are summoned into responsible ways of loving.

To our homosexual brothers and sisters we offer a concluding word. This message has been an outstretched hand to your parents and families, inviting them to accept God's grace present in their lives now and to trust in the unfailing mercy of Jesus our Lord. Now we stretch out our hands and invite you to do the same. We are called to become one body, one spirit in Christ. We need one another if we are to "grow in every way into him who is the head, Christ, from whom the whole body, joined and held together by every supporting ligament, with the proper functioning of each part, brings about the body's growth and builds itself up in love" (*Eph.* 4:15–16).

Though at times you may feel discouraged, hurt or angry, do not walk away from your families, from the Christian community, from all those who love you. In you God's love is revealed. You are always our children.

"There is no fear in love . . . Perfect love drive out fear" (1 *Jn.* 4:18).

Observations on the Revised Text of
Always Our Children
Fr. John Harvey

After reading the text of the *Revised Always Our Children* (RAOC), in *Origins*, vol. 28, #7, July 2, 1998, I regard it as a distinct improvement over the flawed October 1, 1997, document, but it is still characterized by a misleading use of terms and by failure to provide specific kinds of guidance for Catholic parents of children with same-sex attractions. I had noted that Bishop Thomas O'Brien, chairman of the Committee on Marriage and the Family, had consulted with the Sacred Congregation of the Faith on the revision, and that the Congregation was "satisfied" with it. I was curious to know what "satisfied" meant, and so I wrote to Rome because I wanted to publish my reservations about the revision. I received a prompt response which said that I was free to do so.

In his introduction to the revised document, Bishop O'Brien said that "the core message, tone, and direction of *Always Our Children* remains the same as in the first printing." That is precisely why I have reservations about the revision, albeit certain objectionable statements and misuse of Vatican documents, which had appeared in the original, were deleted from it.

I objected strongly to the use of the terms "gay" and "lesbian" in the original document, pointing out that the human person "can hardly be adequately described by a reductionist reference to his or her sexual orientation" (CDF 1986 Letter, sect.16). The terms reappear in the revised document with a caution that they must be used "in honest and accurate ways." The common connotation of the terms "gay" and "lesbian" as understood in the secular media, and as understood by those who label themselves such is that the most important thing about them is their homosexual orientation. The individual will tell you, "This is WHO I AM. I was born this way, and I will always be this way. I intend to live this way. I will find a lover of my own sex with whom I can express my natural sexual feelings."

As long as the individual thinks this way, he is prevented from seeing himself as he really is: a rational creature of God with free will, capable by the grace of God of controlling his sexual desires and, in some instances, as has been empirically established, of getting rid of the condition itself. Each of us is far more than a sexual orientation. Although the revised document acknowledges that "our total personhood is more encompassing than sexual orientation," its acceptance of the terms "gay" and "lesbian" undercuts that very message. Instead of instructing parents to merely "be sensitive to how your son or daughter is using" these terms, it would be better to advise parents to discourage their son or daughter from labeling themselves as "gay" or "lesbian." The 1986 Letter to the Bishops of the Catholic Church carefully avoids these terms, as I have indicated above (sect.16).

My second reservation is concerned with the failure of the revised document to correct its misuse of the 1975 *Declaration on Certain Questions Concerning Sexual Ethics.* The revised document (RAOC) states that "Church teaching acknowledges a distinction between a homosexual tendency that proves to be 'transitory' and 'homosexuals who are definitively such because of some kind of innate instinct.'" It is incorrect to say that this is a matter of Church teaching. In section 8 of *Certain Questions,* the document says that some psychologists hold to this distinction "not without reason." *Certain Questions* repeats the psychological opinion of that time, that some homosexuals "are such because of some kind of innate instinct or because of a constitutional defect presumed to be incurable." Both AOC and RAOC use the phrase "some kind of innate instinct." Such is an erroneous translation of the Latin "quasi-innatus," which should be translated, "as if innate," in other words, not innate. The first Italian edition of the Catholic Catechism which used the word "innate" in describing the homosexual orientation was revised. Explaining the reason, Cardinal

Ratzinger said, "One objection was that we made people think homosexual tendency was innate, that it was already present at the moment of birth or conception of the person. Many competent persons said that this has not been proven." The revised document, however, does not take these points into consideration.

In the paragraph following the reference to *Certain Questions*, RAOC says that we should "understand sexual orientation (homosexual or heterosexual) as a deep-seated dimension of one's personality" and "recognize its relative stability in a person." Equating heterosexual and homosexual in the parenthesis seems to imply that in the view of the *Committee on Marriage and the Family*, heterosexual orientation and homosexual orientation are on the same level – both are "deep-seated" and both have "relative stability."

But heterosexual attraction is natural to man and woman (Catholic *Catechism* #2333), while homosexual tendencies are unnatural, although psychologically understandable. Heterosexual attraction is God-given, and for the vast majority of the human race, leads to marriage, children, and family; same-sex attractions are an objective disorder, but not sinful in themselves (CDF Statement, 1986, sect. 3). The revised document refers to this objective disorder in footnote no.1, but it ought to be explained in the text, as it is in section 3 of the 1986 document. One often hears this objection to the term "objective disorder" being applied to homosexual tendencies: "If a man lusts for a woman or vice versa, this too is an objective disorder." But this is not so, because, if the man or woman controls this natural attraction, and wills to express it in the natural state of marriage, it is a good thing, desired by the Creator. But if one has a sexual-genital attraction to another person of the same sex, it can never lead to a morally good act between the two individuals, but rather it will *always* lead to an immoral act. That is why it is called an objective disorder.

The revised document repeats that it is "a common opinion of experts that there are multiple factors, genetic, hormonal, psychological, that may give rise to homosexual orientation." But there is no "common opinion" among experts on genetic or hormonal factors, and certainly many schools of thought on psychological factors. This document, moreover, does little to distinguish carefully between personal identity and sexual orientation. Our uniqueness as persons is not rooted in our sexual inclinations, but in other intellectual, volitional and bodily characteristics. Our personhood is much more complex than our sexual identity. To center personal identity in a homosexual inclination is to accept a false identity. It may be said that a homosexual orientation is not part of one's uniqueness as a rational or Christian person.

Advice to Parents

The revised documents' advice to parents needs further clarification. It is still not clear whether "child" refers to an adolescent or an adult. In practice, the approach that parents should take toward an adolescent is radically different from the way they relate to a grown son or daughter. It is said that parents should not "presume that your child has developed a homosexual orientation." Then, at the end of the following paragraph, parents are advised to "remain open to the possibility that your son or daughter is struggling to understand and accept a basic homosexual orientation." The use of the term "basic" in this context connotes a fixed condition. This may not be the case, especially in a young person.

Granted it is wise to advise parents not to presume that their child has a homosexual orientation, as well as to prepare the parents for the possibility that their child does struggle with such feelings; however, to refer to such feelings as a "basic homosexual orientation" is problematic. There is no reason why an adolescent should resign himself or herself to "accepting a basic homosexual orientation," even while acknowledging that same-sex attractions are present. Instead, parents should send the adolescent to a reliable therapist who believes in the Catholic teaching on homosexuality for guidance, and later to an experienced priest for counsel.

When it comes to the question of how parents relate to the grown son or daughter who claims to be "gay" or "lesbian," it is important to consider factors not mentioned in the revised document. From many years of counseling such parents, I have learned that in most instances, the grown son or daughter has made up his

225

or her mind to live in a relationship with a same-sex partner. Parents are then faced with a difficult decision whether to approve this relationship or to say to their grown child: "I love you, but I cannot approve your behavior. Please do not ask me to do so." And the usual reply is: "If you love me, you will accept our loving relationship, which for us is like your marriage. But if you do not accept us in our union, then you do not love me." Oftentimes, the grown child will refuse to communicate with his parents. This tragic situation led other Courage members and priests to form Encourage, a spiritual support group in which parents seek pastoral guidance and support for themselves.

Additional Concerns about the Revised Document

1. The revised document does not specify the kinds of retreats that would benefit Catholic parents of adolescents with same-sex attractions, that is to say, retreats in which the retreat master and the Catholic psychologists involved are known for their loyalty to the magisterial teaching of the universal Church. I have known of retreats for Catholic parents of children with same-sex attractions where PFLAG leaders (Parents and Friends of Lesbians and Gays) advised the parents how to respond to adolescent or adult children. PFLAG seeks to persuade parents to accept their children in the sense of accepting the lifestyle of the children. This organization sees homosexual orientation as natural and good in those individuals who identify themselves as "gay" or "lesbian." Parents are told they should accept such persons and their behavior as good and natural, especially in the context of a "faithful" relationship. Such advice is painfully seductive, especially in the case of young persons who are confused about their sexual inclinations.

2. In outlining the various emotional responses of parents who learn that their son or daughter has same-sex attractions, one should include these under the heading FEAR: "You may fear for the spiritual welfare of your child who is active in the homosexual lifestyle." From my dialogue with such parents, I know this is a real concern for them.

3. It is not enough to seek a therapist who "has an appreciation of religious values." The therapist should respect the moral teaching of the Catholic Church on homosexuality. The therapist should be open to the possibility that a young person may be able to move beyond homosexual attractions toward heterosexual development, despite the opposition of the psychological establishment.

4. Under the pastoral recommendations to parents included in AOC, it should be clearly stated (in point number 2) that, while demonstrating love for the child, parents should stand opposed to any kind of homogenital activity, not only because they find it "objectionable," but also because it is seriously immoral.

5. Under AOC's pastoral recommendations to Church ministers, point number 5, the advice to them to seek agencies that "operate in a manner consistent with Church teaching" needs clarification. It should be made clear that the agencies recommended should be faithful to the magisterial teachings of the Church regarding the immorality of homogenital acts. Some agencies sin by omission in that they stress the issue of discrimination, while neglecting the need for a program to promote chastity among persons with same-sex attractions.

6. The advice to seek help from "special diocesan gay and lesbian ministries" is also cause for concern, as our experience has shown that such "ministries" do not provide a program for chaste living. Such programs tend to encourage individuals to define their personhood by their homosexual attractions, labeling themselves according to an objectively disordered inclination.

Conclusion

Once again, we praise the spirit of compassion found in the revised version of *Always Our Children*, and the effort to offer help to every family affected by homosexuality. We hope, however, that a better document can be developed. Members of Courage/ EnCourage pray that the *Committee on Marriage and the Family* will be open to further revisions of this document for the common good of all those persons with same-sex attractions who desire to live faithfully by the teachings of our Catholic Faith.